Transcending Addiction
and
Other Afflictions

Second Edition

Transcending Addiction
and
Other Afflictions

Second Edition

Angela Browne-Miller, PhD, DSW, MPH

Metaterra® Publications

metaterra®
publications

TRANSCENDING ADDICTIONS AND OTHER AFFLICTIONS:
LIFE HEALING

Second Edition

Published in the United States by Metaterra® Publications.
www.Metaterra.com
Library of Congress Cataloging-in-Publication Data.
Browne-Miller, Angela.
Transcending Addiction and Other Afflictions/Angela Browne-Miller – 2nd Edition.
1. Psychology. 2. Social Work 3. Browne-Miller, Angela.
4. Consciousness. 5. Spirituality. 6. Addiction. 7. Substance Abuse.
8. Gambling. 9. Eating Disorders. 10. Depression. 11. Alcoholism.
Title:
TRANSCENDING ADDICTIONS AND OTHER AFFLICTIONS:
LIFE HEALING
Second Edition
Library of Congress Control Number: (see website listed above)
ISBN-13: 978-1-937951-09-2 (Paperback)
ISBN-13: 978-1-937951-10-8 (Kindle ebook)
Published in the United States of America for US and worldwide distribution.
Metaterra® Publications, 1 Blackfield Dr 343, Tiburon, CA 94920, USA.
Cover and content illustrations by and copyright ©Angela Browne-Miller.
Book design by and copyright ©Angela Browne-Miller.
Note: Transcending Addiction and Other Afflictions, first edition, (0893919004 and 0893919039), also copyright Angela Browne-Miller.
Ordering information and bulk ordering information available through:
Amazon Paperback and Amazon Kindle.
Also contact Info@Metaterra.com.

dedicated
to
humanity

NOTE TO READERS:

Thank you for visiting these pages. You will find that the first edition of this book is contained right here, within this second edition. This allows the author's additional thinking to frame the central and ongoing teachings of the basic *Transcending Addiction*. An introduction to the expanded thinking of this second edition is presented in some depth in the first chapter listed below. Note that this first chapter, *Taking Addiction Theory to the Next Level,* contains the author's newest perspectives on and essential understandings of both drug and nondrug addictions. The following is a list of the new chapters and sections created for this second edition:

Taking Addiction Theory to the Next Level: Foreword (to this Second Edition of) Transcending Addiction and Other Afflictions;

Prologue: It is Never Too Late;

Appendix One: Survival and Counter-Survival;

Appendix Two: Need, Desire, Pleasure, Stimulation, and Risk;

Appendix Three: Calling for Complete Overhaul;

Appendix Four: Illustrations.

Table of Contents

Table of Illustrations

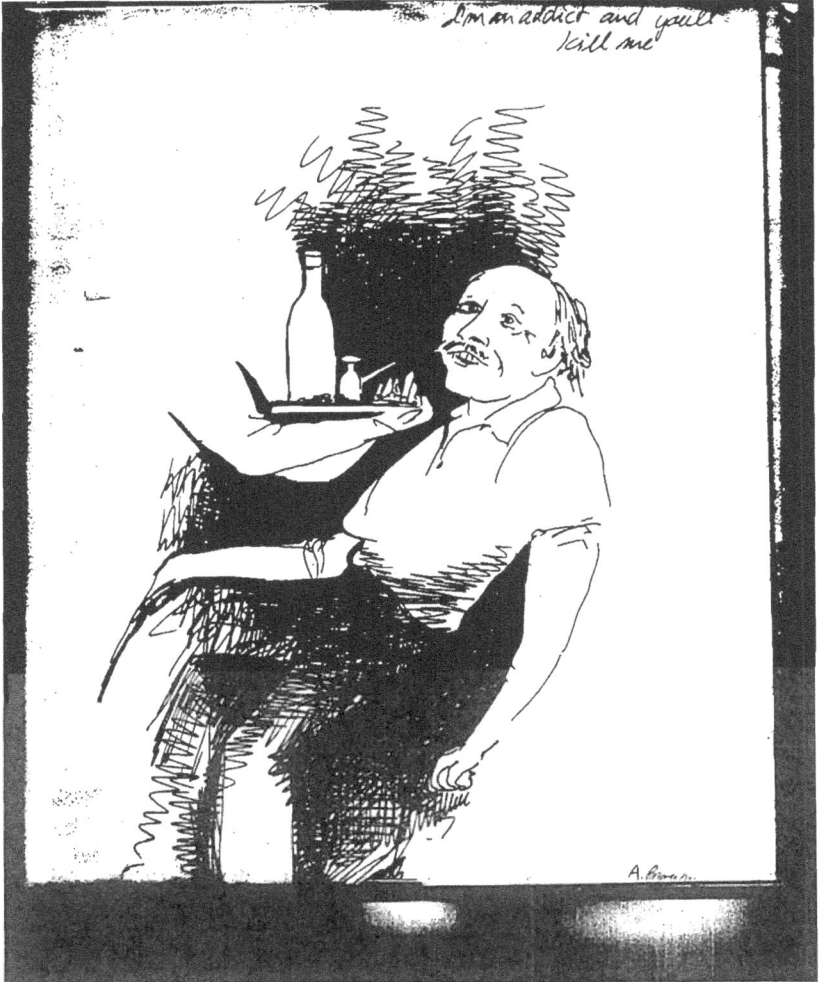

**We Have Seen the Addict
And He Is Us**
(Illustration by and courtesy of Angela Browne-Miller.)

Taking Addiction Theory To the Next Level:

Foreword to
Transcending Addiction
Second Edition

by
Angela Browne-Miller

As if a photo being developed and coming into focus in an old fashioned dark room, the theme of this book becomes increasingly clear as time progresses. *Transcending Addiction*, this book and its theme, have been and continue to be on a long and amazing journey since the first edition of this book was released years ago (at what some say was the inception of the modern perspective on addiction and addiction treatment).

I have had the privilege of walking the journey of the addiction(s) field as it has evolved in our modern times. And I have had the honor of walking with many individuals as they proceeded and now continue to proceed through addiction, and recovery from addiction, and on into what I call the "discovery stage."

And what an immense journey this has been and is. Walking with someone, or with oneself, through profound personal change is a trek of phenomenal distance, every second itself another whole journey.

Prior to the release of that very first edition of *Transcending Addiction*, I indeed had had the honor of working with many persons experiencing drug and nondrug addictions, other afflictions of habit and compulsion, and various emotional and physical cycles appearing to have no real exit. It was quite clear to me that the sometimes visible and sometimes invisible journeys these persons were making were highly intense and truly remarkable for them and for those around them – including for me.

Since the release of that first edition of *Transcending Addiction*, I have worked with thousands more persons seeking to shift their patterns of behavior, to break their problem additions and other afflictions. I have seen thousands of persons rewire themselves, rewrite their patterns, shifting from problem patterns to productive ones. These days, the notion that a pattern of behavior, an emotion, and or an energy circuit can be rewired, even transcended, is central in my work.

What becomes ever more clear is that we are all at risk for problem patterning, for acquiring many so-called "bad" habits and developing sometimes severe addictions. Some of the most obvious mild, moderate, problem, and severe addictions are those to substances: alcohol, nicotine, and other drugs. Yet, it is not only substances that can be addicting. It is also attitudes, emotions, relationships to people and to things, and other behaviors that can be addicting. Furthermore, although already obvious to me at the time of the writing of the first edition of this book, it is now ever more clear that the key (biochemical, physical, emotional, cognitive, etc.) roles that implicit, underlying, patterns play in explicit addictions must be well addressed. Otherwise we treat the symptoms – the obvious addictions – without addressing what underlying patterns and behaviors fuel and then perpetuate these addictions. Both my research and my time with my clients have led me to recognize the marked presence and power of underlying programmings behind our explicit habits and addictions.

The work of overcoming detrimental habits and addictions is, in essence, dialoging with the magnificent although perhaps somewhat archaic human brain. Behavioral change, especially the "breaking" (as it is called) of habits and addictions, involves change at the micro and at the macro levels of being, in fact on all levels of being. And virtually all the patterns on these levels are directed by the mind and by its brain (the latter which organizes, drives, and, for the most part, houses control of these patterns). Where we — as addicted or co-addicted persons (which as I explain herein is all of us in some way), or as addiction treatment or other health professionals, or as those who research or legislate addiction — strive to encourage such profound behavioral change, we speak to the human brain virtually every day, virtually every moment of every day.

This book is written with this speaking to the mind-brain in mind. The wording of this material is such that persons in all walks of life, lay and or professional, can access and share the ideas and the presentation of these ideas with themselves and others, including persons who are addicted and co-addicted – and otherwise afflicted -- with problem patterns of personal, familial, social, and species forms -- patterns housed within our genes, and our biologies, biochemistries, neurologies, psychologies, sociologies, and so on. Basically, we must talk to the minds, the individual and the species minds, of the human beings who are experiencing problem addictions and afflictions.

Think of my words as a simple dialog with the mind-brain/s of the individual and of the species, an attempt to befriend the mind-brain, to coax it, to inspire it, into prompting within itself profound behavioral change. After all, communicating in a manner that will be heard is already adjusting the communication process in the direction of increased accessibility.

In working with several thousand persons who are addicted and co-addicted, whether it be to substances or to behaviors—to drugs, alcohol, food, on-ground and online gambling and gaming, online and on-ground sex, relationships themselves, spending and shopping, television, work, violence, and or hundreds of other materials and activities, and millions of problem patterns, I have seen the addict and *I know the addict to be us – all of us*. I see that:

- habits and addictions themselves can be seen as a natural part of life, with many habits and addictions being positive, healthy and some even necessary behaviors;
- detrimental habits and addictions can be identified as such, clearly seen as behavior for which we are naturally coded now gone awry (discussed further in Appendices One, Two and Three at the end of this book);
- troubled and dangerous addictions can be overcome what I term "situationally"; and,
- overcoming detrimental habits and addictions requires a rewiring of ourselves—a rewiring of the self and of its perceptions of its situation—a rewiring of our minds and brains, and of our spirits, to change our behaviors.

Stepping back for a moment, let's turn to another aspect of our functioning, the heart beat. Here is something, a pattern, not only natural to our biological functioning, but essential. And when there is a troubled heart beat, one that may be either mildly troubling or seriously dangerous, we identify this heart beat and where required treat it. However, we do not call the beating of the heart itself a sickness, a disease. And we do not say that heart should not beat.

Hence where we find patterning behavior which brings about addictions and habits, we do not seek to remove that very essential to life patterning behavior. Instead we want to heal problem patterns. We do not need to call the patterning behavior itself a sickness, a disease. Pattern addiction itself, in this larger sense of the word, is not a disease. *Problem addiction* is the disease where disease is the model we are applying. Clearly, we do not need to say that we, the organism, should not become patterned or addicted to "good" patterns such as stopping at red lights, putting on seat belts, brushing teeth, riding a bicycle, (perhaps to even deeper biological patterns and directives such as basic breathing and digesting), and so on.

Now, all this is rather obvious. We are all creatures reliant upon our ability to grow patterned, all even addicted to both positive and likely also negative behaviors. Where we run into problems, very serious problems, is when this patterning capability within us seriously malfunctions (in terms of the survival value of the pattern) either because of internal or external factors: directives, susceptibilities, vulnerabilities, and or pressures on us.

So we are all addicted to many things and to many behaviors, as we are all coded to be. Perhaps even most of what we as individuals, families and societies do in our lives is driven by some form of pattern addiction. We are born with this capacity to be addicted and even need it. No one is exempt. Addiction to patterns is common to all of us. Addiction to situations in which we can play out our patterns is also common to all of us. We even favor—exhibit attentional biases toward—conditions and triggers for these patterns.

In making this second edition of *Transcending Addiction* available now, in these ever more modern times, I want to bring the SELF fully into focus. I want to say that getting to truly know oneself, to really know one's SELF, is to delineate between: (a) the true self; and, (b) the problem pattern addiction that appears to be the self or part of the self, but is not. We are *not* our problem patterns, these are not our identities, although it is easy to err and think these are one in the same. In fact, in my work I have walked with so many problem patterns, looked so many in the eye, that I have come to see how these problem patterns take on a life of their own. They camouflage themselves by assuming the identities of the persons they inhabit.

These problem patterns do most definitely seek to dominate the brains and identities they inhabit, to utilize all attentional, energetic and nutritional resources to sustain, grow and protect themselves. I have seen them doing this. I catch them when working with the people and minds these problem patterns are seeking to take control of.

So now, as the addict, which is all of us, we can reposition ever so slightly our approach to overcoming problem addiction patterns, which is going to also be repositioning rather profoundly. Walk with me now, through the following pages where we can return to the place from which we started, the SELF: knowing this SELF for the first time.

Note: Readers seeking further discussion of the issues raised in this Foreword will please see the Appendices included at the end of this second edition of *Transcending Addiction and Other Afflictions*:

Appendix One: Survival and Counter-Survival;
Appendix Two: Need, Desire, Pleasure, Stimulation, and Risk;
Appendix Three: Calling for Complete Overhaul.

**EXPLICIT (SURFACE) PATTERN ADDICTION
(PRESENTING PROBLEM)**

↑

**IMPLICIT (HIDDEN)
PATTERN ADDICTION**

↑

**UNDERLYING SOURCE
PATTERNING:
PROGRAMMING/CODING
TO BE ADDICTED**

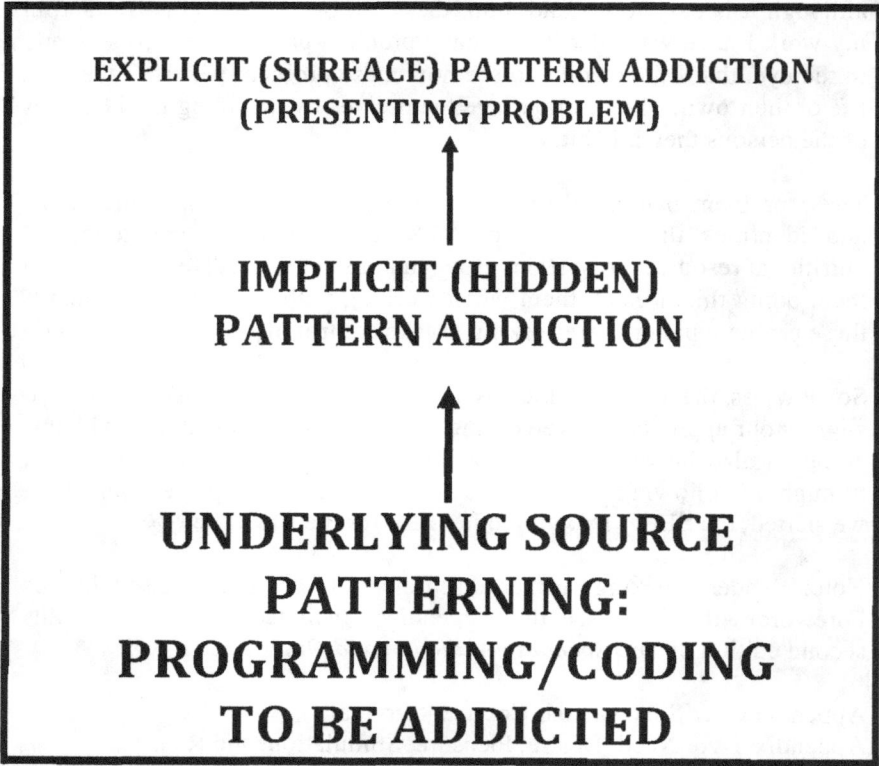

**EVER UNDERLYING SOURCE PATTERNING
AND CODING**
(Illustration by and courtesy of Angela Browne-Miller.)

```
┌─────────────────────────────────────────────────────────────────┐
│                      PERCEIVED ADDICTIVITIES                      │
│                                                                   │
│  <<< CAFFEINE            ALCOHOL          METHAMPHETAMINE>>>       │
│                        (as examples)                              │
│                                                                   │
│  low level of perceived addictivity                               │
│                    ← -------------------------------→             │
│                              high level of perceived addictivity  │
│                                                                   │
│  highly acceptable addiction                                      │
│                    ← -------------------------------→             │
│                              low or no acceptable addiction       │
│                                                                   │
│  low degree of distinguishable harm                               │
│                    ← -------------------------------→             │
│                              high degree of distinguishable harm  │
│                                                                   │
│  highly acceptable harm                                           │
│                    ← -------------------------------→             │
│                              low or no acceptable harm            │
│                                                                   │
│  high tolerance for a particular addiction                        │
│                    ← -------------------------------→             │
│                        low or no tolerance for a particular addiction │
└─────────────────────────────────────────────────────────────────┘
```

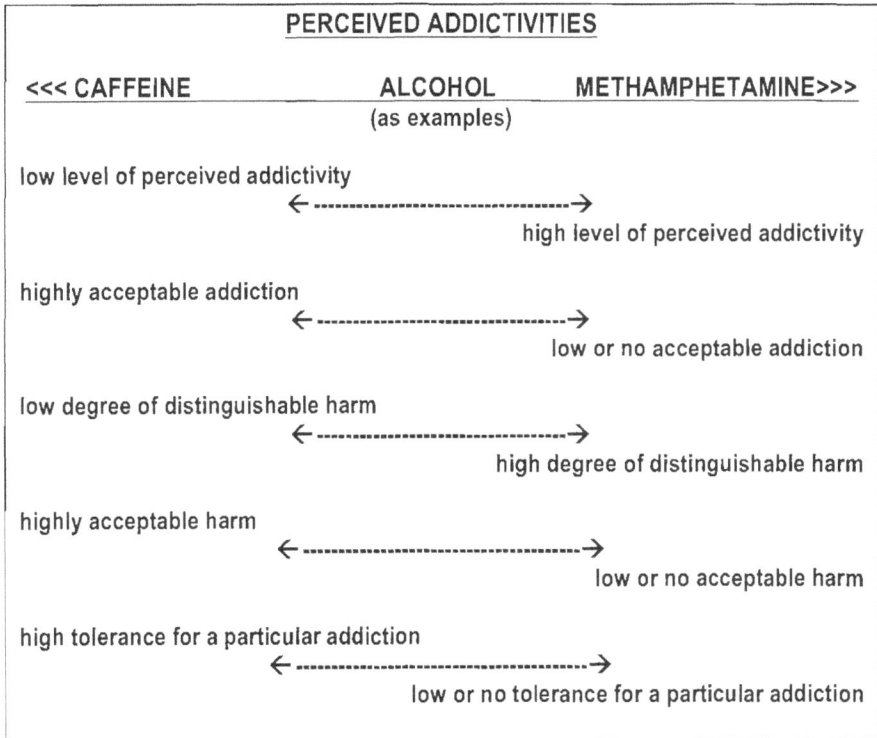

**PERCEPTIONS REGARDING
ADDICTIVITY OF VARIOUS SUBSTANCES VARY**
(Illustration by and courtesy of Angela Browne-Miller.)

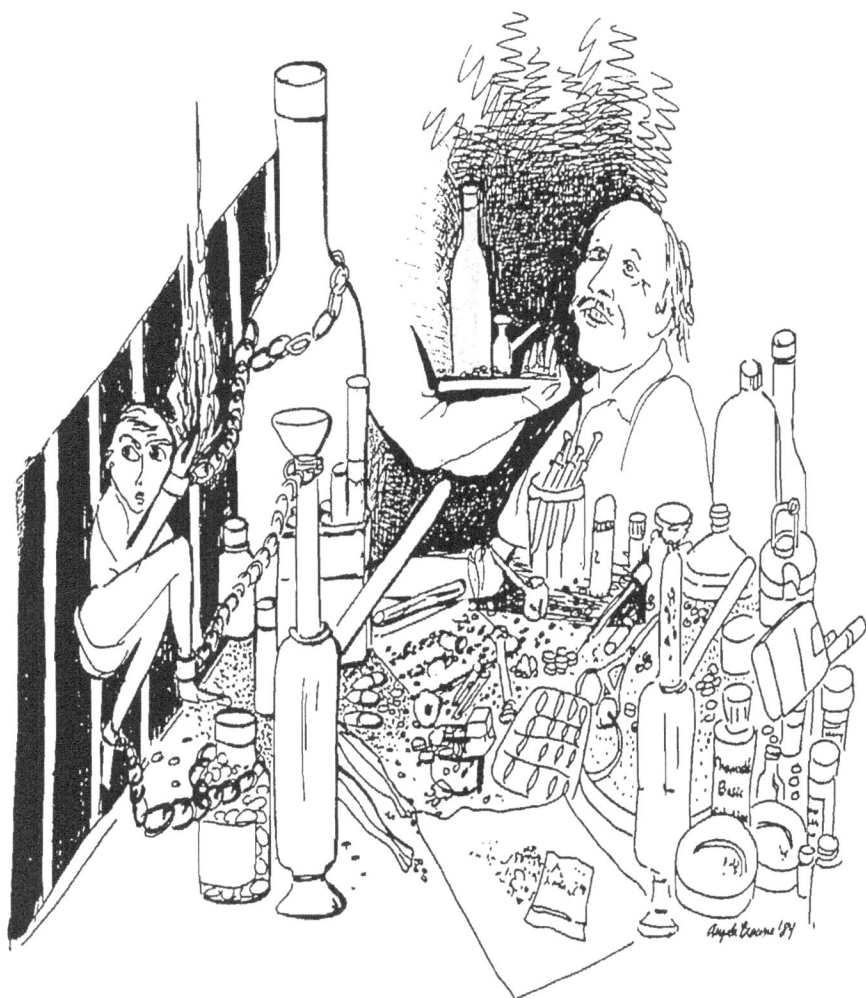

Answer Problem Addiction with Complete Overhaul
(Illustration by and courtesy of Angela Browne-Miller.)

DRUG CATEGORIES AND DRUGS: PARTIAL LIST
(Continued on following page.)

DRUG CATEGORIES
(examples of)

SPECIFIC DRUGS
(examples of)

Narcotics

Alfentanil
Cocaine*
Codeine
Crack Cocaine*
Fentanyl
Heroin
Hydromorphone
Ice
Meperidine
Methadone
Morphine
Nalorphine
Opium
Oxycodone
Propoxyphene

Depressants

Benzodiazepine
Chloral Hydrate
Chlordiazepoxide
Diazepam
Glutethimide
Meprobamate
Methaqualone
Nitrous Oxide
Pentobarbital
Secobarbital

Alcohol

Ethyl Alcohol

Stimulants/Inhalants

Amphetamine
Benzedrine
Benzphetamine
Butyl Nitrite
Dextroamphetamine
Methamphetamine
Methylphenidate
Phenmetrazine

Hallucinogens

Bufotenine
LSD
MDA
MDEA
MDMA
Mescaline
MMDA
Phencyclidine
Psilocybin

Cannabis

Marijuana
Tetrahydrocannabinol

Steroids

Dianabol
Nandrolone

DRUG CATEGORIES AND DRUGS: PARTIAL LIST
(The above is continued from preceding page.)

EXAMPLES OF NONDRUG ADDICTIONS
(Note: This is only a partial list of non-substance addictions.)

Gambling Addiction	On-Ground, Direct Telephone On-Line, Internet
Gaming Addiction	On-Ground, Direct Telephone On-Line, Internet
Sex Addiction	On-Ground, Direct Telephone On-Line, Internet
Pornography Addiction	On Ground, Direct Telephone On-Line, Internet
Relationship Addiction	On Ground, Direct Telephone On-Line, Internet
Eating	Compulsive Eating, All Foods Compulsive Eating, Carbohydrates Compulsive Eating, Other Specific Food Groups Overeating Undereating, Annorexia Bulemia
Self-Mutilation	Cutting, Mutillating Burning, Bruising
Work Addiction	Long Work Hours Large Workloads
Television Addiction	Long Viewing Hours
Abuse & Violence Against Others	Abuse, Forms of Violence, Forms of

(Chart by and courtesy of Angela Browne-Miller.)

Prologue:
It Is Never Too Late

It is never, never, too late. You find yourself struggling in the rubble of broken dreams. You have been there a moment, a month, a decade — however long. You may feel your pain, your tears, your sense of loss and hopelessness, or you may just feel confusion, or you may just feel nothing at all. You say please, please some one fix this. Please please show me a way out. Please please God, if you are out there, help me.

The bits and pieces of the life you wanted to lead lie around you, shattered. You may weep or you may scream or you may sit in numb silence. You tread carefully through the fragments of your fractured dreams because you hurt when you walk on them, as if they are broken glass and your feet are bare. Everywhere you see wasteland, your own personal wasteland.

But these bits are the ingredients of something new. Put them together like pieces of a jigsaw puzzle, and you will solve the mystery of the new you. There is a secret there among those ruins, there is something new waiting for you to see: There is always time to begin again . . . .

A hand reaches out from somewhere, a hand you can almost see. Is it your imagination or is there someone there? Look again, the hand you see is your own. Yes, there may be others trying to help. Or you may be all alone in this. But the hand you see is your own. You are calling yourself back to life. Listen. You want to be heard. You want to come back.

The view from this rock bottom place is the best view ever. Open your eyes. From here you can truly see. The possibilities are endless. Believe that you can resurrect yourself — believe — and you can.

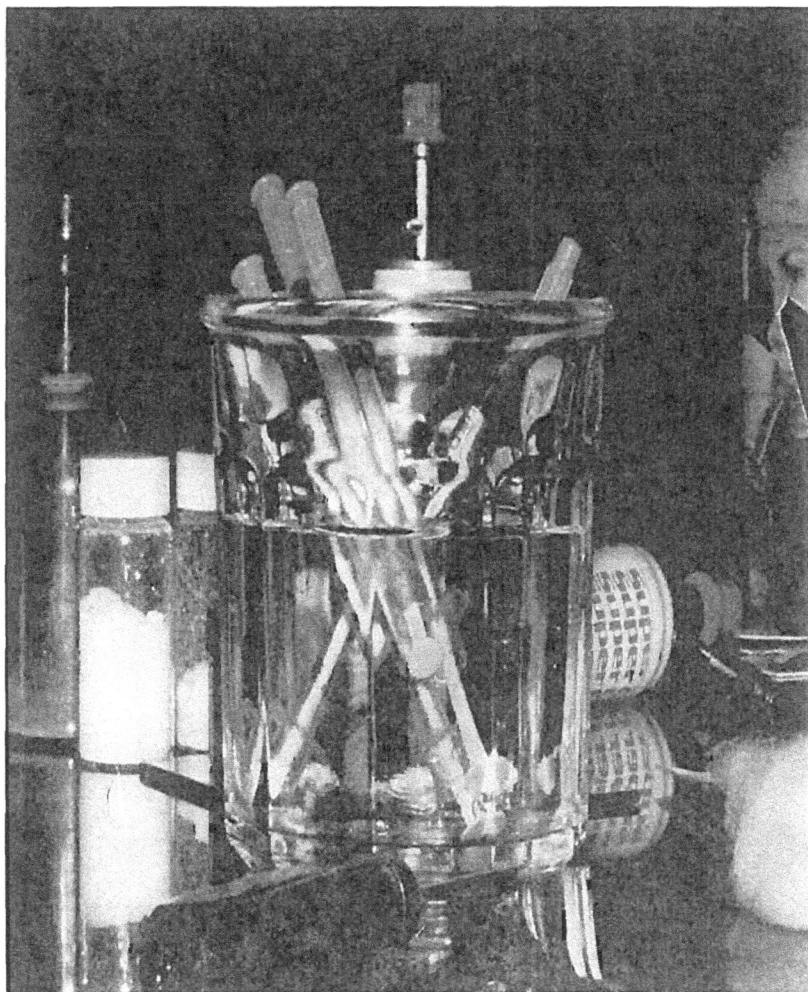

Overcome Problem Addictions Around and Within
(Photograph by and courtesy of Angela Browne-Miller.)

xxx

Introduction:
Death and Transcendence

$\mathbf{A}$re we biological, fleshy robots? Do we reflect a sallow mechanical light in our eyes, the light of willessness, the glow of hypnotization? Have we succumbed to a daze in modern years or have we always been part of a very large mindlessness—are we biotech at its finest? Or biotech gone wrong?

If earth is a fantastic macrocosmic laboratory and we are prisoner-subjects in a massive experiment too large for our human minds to fathom, then our transcendences can lead to startling discoveries regarding our captors. Perhaps we can capture control of our wills and set them free. But what would this freedom look like? Would it be much different than the way we live and look now? Can we really be free as long as we are subject to the enslavement of inherited and acquired, genetic and neurological, programming?

These are questions more readily asked than answered. Yet we might move toward an inkling of an answer if we reflect upon the degrees of freedom allowed us by biology. Consider the view that we function on genetic and neurological automatic the majority of the time. We fool ourselves into believing that we exercise a great deal of free will. We are in a state of denial about our mechanical, robotic, programmed, and programmable nature.

We living things are creatures of habit. Our ability to biologically (and even genetically) program ourselves for automatic responses is essential for survival. Speedy responses to danger, for example, save lives. If we had to take time to think through each action, we'd probably die off. We rely on our automatic behaviors to respond to physical events such as falling objects, red traffic lights and other situations that demand a quick response. We also may respond automatically to seemingly less critical physical events or conditions such as hunger for a snack, a cold draft in the house, or a baby's cry. Some pieces of this behavior are genetically inherited and thus instinct driven, and other pieces are the result of patterning acquired during day-to-day experiences.

So convenient and readily developed is automatic physical behavior that it merges with the nonphysical realms of human interaction and emotion. Public and private feelings, and their expressions, are often manifestations of psychological and social patterns. It is difficult to discern exactly what proportion of an individual's behavior is attributable to the larger social and cultural environment, and what proportion is particular, idiosyncratic to the individual.

This ambiguity is especially true in cases of food and drug addiction. So much of our cultural overlay is dedicated to the selling and feeding of food and at least legal drugs to the consumer. We are bombarded by advertisements to eat food, drink alcohol, and smoke cigarettes. Is overconsumption, or addiction to any of these or similar drugs, merely an individual malady, or is it an acquired response to environmental stimulation? And even if this question could be definitively answered, there is still the matter of programming. Once a behavior, no matter what its origin, is repeated a number of times, a program is eroded into the neural pathways that have transmitted the biochemical message required to repeat the act. The more repetition, the deeper the erosion, the more automatic the behavior. The robot within us rises, run by automatic programming, at once the prison and the prisoner of life. Meet the biological robot: You, me, everyone.

There is no way, except perhaps death, to clear the mind of all past impressions and programming. Those who believe in the spillover of experience from lifetime to lifetime will claim that even death is not a clearing. But let us say, for argument's sake, that biological death is an effective means of erasure, and that only death offers complete erasure. Death, then, is a sure means of overcoming or transcending a problematic personal condition, especially if the problem condition is, as are most conditions of human behavior, subject to neurological and other forms of biological patterning. Death, under appropriate circumstances, is an honorable option.

Or maybe death is not a complete erasure but, instead, a sort of amnesia, allowing whatever it is that may live on when the body dies a chance to forget its biological programming. What a marvelous opportunity this might be for those who are deeply dissatisfied with the programming that they have either inherited or acquired. But we cannot be certain that all deaths guarantee transcendence. It is therefore as important to die well as it is to live well. Preparation for death is preparation for transcendence.

While I stand in favor of an individual's right to choose death, I am not advocating physical death to as the only way out of problem conditions. I have seen too many lives turn around, too many healings and recoveries, to believe that there is no way except physical death to escape those conditions. Physical death is merely one category of death along a continuum, or a matrix, of deaths. Death, whatever form it may take, offers the opportunity for transcendence, but in no way guarantees it. Again it is important to die well, whether or not the death in question is biological. Death can be lifehealing.

Transcendence may occur spontaneously in death; however, it may be more likely to occur with adequate preparation. In this sense, all of life can be preparation for death; and, several deaths may occur within one's lifetime. If we think of death as the shedding of old programming and of biological life as the acquiring of new programming, then biological death appears to be the shedding of old neurological, biochemical, and genetic skin—and other forms of death offer the shedding of at least some of the same. Death appears to be a route to freedom, or at least to an increase in degrees of freedom. This increase lasts only as long as new programming is resisted and old programming is not rediscovered.

The latter possibility deserves our critical attention. It appears that we become *addicted to the very programming* we would shed in death, and that we resist this shedding. We tend to resist death, in whatever form this transformation may take, just as addicted people are driven (by this programming) to resist shedding the desires for the drugs or the objects of their addictions. When this shedding finally takes place, death occurs as a healing event.

In accord with this line of thought, and by the above definitions, only soul death (experienced by the dead soul) fails to involve true death. What I call *soul death* is the surrender of the soul to the mechanical, the programmable self. Soul death is actually the refusal to die—the refusal to shed the automatic mechanical side of one's self.

Too many of us respond to this concept by saying, "Well then, I am not a dead soul. I am much too feeling, too emotional, to be one." This is an error in perception. When feelings are vented, expressed, as part of a repeating emotional pattern or program, no matter how dramatic the feelings may be, they are robotic, mechanical, and predictable as an action–reaction formula. This is, for some, a difficult concept to absorb, because we have been taught that the expression of emotion is the opposite of the absence of that expression.

Think, instead, in terms of patterns. Breaking out of a pattern (a habit of emotion or of action or of energy or of illness or of drug use or of gambling, etc.) is the opposite of being addicted to a pattern. Breaking a pattern is dying. Are you prepared to die? Are you prepared to release old patterns? Are you ready to transcend? Will you succeed? Can you die well?

To do so, you must break your addiction to the programming that controls, or in some way relates to, the pattern you are talking about breaking. What is offered in this book is a recipe for transcendence of one's programming. I use drug and alcohol addiction as a primary example, because this is an area in which the problem of programming is most obvious. Those concerned about painful relationship patterns, chronic pain, life-threatening diseases, and other crises of one's programming are working with the same question—how does one break out of one's addiction to one's programming? What type of death will you require to release—to free—yourself? The only difference between the obvious and the more hidden pattern addictions is that some addictions to programming are more subtle than others. The drug-addicted individual sees a physical thing, a drug, to which he or she is addicted. Individuals dealing with repeated emotional or physical health patterns often have no physical objects onto which they can project or externalize their patterns. This makes the problem-process of addiction to one's programming much more difficult to see, more implicit.

The first step, then, is to face the addiction to patterns in all of us. In this, explicit addictions serve as great learning vehicles. They make the components of pattern addiction much more apparent to us. Implicit addictions are often discovered by people who are in recovery from explicit addictions or who are fighting serious physical illnesses. These individuals become examples for all of us. They lead the way through the matrix of death into the realm of transcendence.

Part I

Facing the Addiction
In All of Us

You will know the truth and the truth will make you free.
—Jesus Christ, John 8:32

1

Addiction as a Model of Affliction

This book is about far more than drug addiction. It is about addiction to any form of destructive or dangerous pattern. Throughout, I refer to what I call *implicit* and *explicit addictions*. Explicit addictions are the more obvious, visible addictions. Overeating, drug and alcohol dependence, and gambling tend to be easily recognized or explicit addictions. Yet these are, basically, only symptoms of more implicit addictions to behavioral, emotional and energetic patterns. And detrimental pattern addiction, even when life threatening, does not always signal its presence through explicit addictions. It can be very difficult to detect.

Pattern addiction is part of the human condition. The more prepared we are to detect and transcend detrimental patterns, the more active a role we can play in our emotional, physical, and spiritual health.

Pattern addiction frequently manifests itself in explicit symptoms such as drug addiction, physical pain, chronic ailments including ulcers, and even cancer. Implicit pattern addictions are built over a long period of time. This is because most neurological programming, the establishment of electrical or energetic patterns throughout the body, takes place over time. Such patterning becomes detrimental when harmful to the emotional, physical, and or spiritual well-being of the individual (or family or community). Some pattern addiction is so subtle, so very implicit, that it involves holding patterns or blockages of necessary electrical charges, full blood flow, and ample oxygen to remote parts of the body. By *remote,*

I mean nerve endings, organs, and other tissues of which we are often unaware. For example, tight musculature surrounding digestive organs can interfere with the transmission of oxygen and neurological impulses involved in building or using digestive enzymes. Tight musculature in the head and neck can lead to jaw grinding. As Oriental medicine suggests, most afflictions are the product of energy flow disturbances. A rebalancing or correction in the transmission of neurological energy throughout the body can alleviate many health problems. When this rebalancing (which is often difficult to achieve) occurs, a harmful energetic pattern, an implicit pattern addiction, is broken. All too often, medicine treats the explicit symptoms of an affliction—the physical pain, the ulcer, the tumor, the drug addiction—without correcting the underlying and more implicit pattern addictions, the programming behind the symptoms. This is, of course, due in part to the inability of current medical technology to do more.

Drug addiction offers one of the most tangible examples of patterning and some of the most tangible evidence that addiction to a pattern can be transcended. I therefore select drug addiction as my primary, but not only, example in this book. You will see the parallels between drug addiction and all pattern addiction.

Let's examine the societal implications of this most threatening explicit addiction of modern times. (I include alcohol whenever I refer to drugs.) Many illusions surround drug and alcohol addiction. One is the illusion of health. Far too many addicted individuals are in a state of denial about their health problems. Too many claim that they are not addicted and use their seemingly good health as proof that they are not addicted. But their lives are wounded. These people are operating under the *illusion* of health as well as under the *illusion* of not being addicted. Most people who suffer from any sort of pattern addiction are in a state of denial about its severity, if they admit its existence at all.

It's not only the addicted individual who generates illusions; much of the addiction treatment and medical community operates under the *illusion* that addiction requires "treatment" and that the forms of medical treatment provided are appropriate for treating addiction. Pattern addiction, however, is not a symptom that can be medicated; it is not a tumor that can be cut out; it is not a sickness that can be fully treated by traditional medical practices. Addiction is a crisis of the heart and soul. But in that crisis lies the possibility of transformation. (*Transformation* and *transcendence* are not typical listings in the medical school curriculum.)

Crisis is opportunity—opportunity for attention. Most people wait for a major psychological or physical crisis to begin to even vaguely address their pattern addictions. For drug addicted persons, this crisis is called *hitting bottom.* Hitting bottom can compel addicted or otherwise afflicted individuals to seize the opportunity to learn—and care—about their mental, physical, and spiritual health. Hitting bottom is a call to action. Many people who think that they have never been detrimentally pattern addicted have not experienced this opportunity. Because the process of overcoming deep pattern addiction requires change on all levels, addiction can actually provide a rare opportunity for profound personal change, and for the realization of one's psychological, creative, and spiritual potentials.

Today, at least some members of the addiction treatment community have come to understand that the *crisis of addiction* provides the *opportunity for transformation.* Effective addiction treatment is not "warehousing" the unwanted or incompetent members of society. It is not "protecting sick people from themselves," or even "protecting society from sick people." It is important for the health care community (of which the addiction treatment community is a part) to recognize addiction and all forms of afflictions as opportunities for transformation, and to seek to bring about that transformation. When addicted or ill individuals arrive at a treatment service, program, or facility, they should find themselves at the door to mental, physical, and spiritual health. Only then will they stand on the threshold of *transcendence.*

All too often, addicted and otherwise afflicted individuals find themselves standing at a door to anything but health. Drug treatment, and most health care services, manifest a range of attitudes toward affliction, but they rarely say, "Welcome. We are fortunate to have you among us, because you are about to lead us in an exploration of the mind, body and spirit. You are about to meet the challenge of addiction to patterning and through that challenge explore the frontiers of healing, of freedom, of human potential, and of the human soul. We are truly fortunate to have you among us."

Instead, addicted people are stigmatized, frowned upon, punished, or treated "like sick people," and "sick people" are treated as society's unwanted. It is not so much a lack of expertise that is the problem with most health care, it is a lack of understanding: understanding what "sick" individuals are all about and respect for the critical role that they play in the evolution of human consciousness.

We have heard so much about "the drug problem" in recent years. Indeed, drug addiction is a crisis, not only for the addicted individual, but for everyone in our society. However, we need to better understand this crisis. It signals the tension in two major areas of modern existence. One is the problem of *chemicalization.* Slowly, manmade chemicals are filling our air, our water, our food, our bodies, and our minds. Our homes are cleaned with detergents. Plastics are everywhere—we wear them, we play with them, we even drive them. Medicine offers chemical solutions to many of our health problems. A reliance on contrived chemicals has become a way of life in our modern world. As a result, we are all becoming chemically dependent. Drug- and alcohol-addicted people are making the reality of everyone's increasing dependence on chemicals more apparent.

The second area of tension is caused by the problem of *mechanization*. Slowly, almost invisibly, we are surrendering our individual freedom. We are acquiescing to the reality of what I call *numbership*—a reality in which we identify ourselves as a series of numbers (telephone, social security, drivers licence, tax identification, etc.) and mechanical processes (checking in and checking out, registering, paying, driving, etc.). Without even seeing it happen, we are beginning to treat ourselves as machines. It is ironic that contained in the word *numbership* is the word *numb*. As we become more like machines, we actually become numb to our humanity. Many addicted individuals claim that they want to "numb the pain" of their existences by using drugs to "turn off." We are learning to turn ourselves on and off with switches. Some of us use chemical switches, and some of us are addicted to the chemical switches we call "drugs." It may be more than just some of us. Just about everyone has turned to painkillers to deal with headaches, body aches, and injuries. Check the inside of your medicine chest. Can you toss out its contents without hesitation?

Chemical switches are part of modern (and maybe ancient) life. And so are electrical switches (such as television) and emotional switches (such as events we rely upon to change our feelings, i.e., parties for energy or happiness, music for sexual arousal or relaxation, holidays for loneliness or comfort, disagreements for anger or righteousness, full blown arguements for violence or tension release). As you can see from this partial list, the switches are not, in themselves, bad for us. It is the way we use them and the tendency we have to rely on them—to run on automatic— rather than to pay attention to how we are turning events, objects, and chemicals into switches and ourselves into things that can be switched on and off.

Because of our shared dependence upon switches, we can see that the drug addiction treatment community has the opportunity to turn the social crises of chemicalization and mechanization into opportunities for everyone. If the treatment community can turn chemicalization and mechanization around in the individuals it treats, then it can make an impact on the societal level as well. Society is made up of individuals, some of whom manifest explicit addictions, and all of whom are subject to implicit addictions that may be harmful. Addiction treatment can become the door to individual *and* to societal health, especially if that treatment can expand to include implicit addiction. Some of this implicit addiction will be what medicine has been calling chronic and acute illness. We all must make way for a change of thought about all forms of what we call *disease* and the medical community is no exception.

As you read on in this book, remember that, when I refer to *drug addiction*, I am including alcohol as a drug. Also keep in mind that the principles of transcendence apply equally well to any kind of destructive dependence, whether on drugs, food, work, another person, an idea, a feeling, or a blood flow or energy pattern. The exercises described herein can be easily adapted to serve your own and or your own patients' needs. Study groups and seminars can be formed to assist readers of this book in applying and understanding the techniques I describe.

Note also that this book can be especially valuable as an accompaniment to other forms of help that an afflicted person may need, including prayer, psychotherapy, self-help meetings, and health care. The concepts and exercises offered herein are intended to serve as an adjunct to the help that is available rather than to entirely replace it. I seek to provoke thought, self-examination, and new ideas about mental and physical illnesses on the individual and, ultimately, the societal level. Join me now in this exploration.

2

We Have Seen the Addict and He Is Us: A Study of Explicit Drug Addiction

When a society, a globe full of societies, grows alarmed about drug trafficking, narcoterrorism, and drug addiction, it is responding to explicit problems. And yet there is an unspoken, intuitive understanding of the implicit spiritual ramifications of such explicit problems. Something about the deepest level of the human condition is being expressed.

In recent years our government has conducted a much-publicized "war on drugs." Besides cracking down on drug dealers and closing our borders to drug smugglers, this "war" has consisted primarily of a variety of television spots describing the dangers of drug and alcohol abuse. There is little convincing evidence that this campaign was highly successful. Although information about the dangers of mind- and body-altering chemicals is helpful, it is not enough to cure addiction. We don't need television to tell us that drugs and alcohol are harmful. Chemically dependent people are not drawn to truth but to satisfy their cravings. The chemically dependent world may not be drawn to truth either.

CONCEPTS OF ADDICTION

The problem of addiction goes much deeper than a simple lack of knowledge or a failure of border closure. Chemical dependence is only one expression of a far more common and more harmful behavior that afflicts our society—destructive dependence. Anyone can fall into a destructive habit. Some people have a destructive dependence on food, others on sex, still others on the people in their close personal relationships—and some people have a destructive chemical dependence. The reality of human existence is that a "little addict person" lurks within all of us. To better understand this little addict person we all share, let's consider two key concepts: *addictive materialism* and *addictive inadequacy*. These are most readily understood in cases of tangible addiction, because tangible or explicit addiction patterns are more easily traced than more subtle explicit patterns, which may or may not have overt physical expression.

Addictive Materialism

One way to look at explicit addiction is to see drug- and/or object-addicted people as materialistic. They reach outside themselves for a material thing—a sort of mechanism—a car, a house, someone's body, food, or, in this case, a drug—as a way of working with their psyches. For example, if they feel depressed, they may take "a drink," a "hit," or "a line." They depend upon an external material item to rescue them from an undesired internal state of mind. Of course their state of mind may reflect external predicaments—things going on in the world around them—but their ability to cope with those predicaments is not based on a continual process of interacting with those predicaments. Instead it is naively based on a concrete external item or object, usually to be taken or experienced physically, as in a "line" or "drink." The addicted individual's preoccupation with a chemical substance is an escape from the more arduous task of really dealing with feelings and situations. Drugs have become the "answer" for so many of us. In a materialistic society, we are conditioned to depend on a material substance in order to avoid the pain of actually living through and learning from a crisis.

Addictive Inadequacy

During the 1960s, young drug users claimed that they were "turning on" and "raising their consciousnesses" through the use of mind-altering chemicals. A few decades later, it has become clear that many of these users, perhaps without even being aware of it, were actually trying to turn *off* and to *diminish* their consciousnesses. This kind of user has come to rely on drugs (including alcohol) to take the more jagged edges off the harsh realities of life. In this picture of drug addiction, individuals use drugs, not because of their material characteristics, but simply because they cannot cope. Their psychological coping mechanisms are insufficient and inadequate in the face of the pressures of modern life. Most of us are taught adequate coping skills as we grow up in this society. But if chemically addicted individuals have learned any of these skills, they lose them through disuse when they handicap themselves with the artificial coping mechanisms of alcohol and other drugs.

These two explanations point to the global nature of explicit addiction. The problems of addictive materialism (dependence on outer means for solving inner problems) and of addictive inadequacy (an inadequate internal coping mechanism) are common to a greater portion of society than the mere population of those addicted to chemicals. How many of us go shopping and end up overspending when we are bored, depressed or faced with a crisis? How many of us have trouble dealing with the realities of life and are forced to depend on externalities? Not all of us are addicted to dangerous chemicals, but we all exhibit signs of addictive materialism and addictive inadequacy. Each of us regularly seeks to compensate for these addictive characteristics within ourselves. This means that the addicted individual is not alone, and not unlike the seemingly nonaddicted person. We all have a great deal in common. If we are honest with ourselves we will admit that we have seen the addict. And he, or she, is us.

Clearly understanding the universal nature of addiction teaches us a lot about how the problem of drug abuse can happen to "people just like us," and even to ourselves. People in trouble with drugs are everyday, regular people whose addictive tendencies have somehow fallen into one of the most dangerous of dependencies.

It's easy to say, "But those addicted people are different from me. I could never do that. And no one in my family could either!" But don't kid yourself. That's what many addicted people and their family members once said.

MOVING TOWARD ADDICTION

Addiction sneaks up on people. Take, for example, the development of a drug addiction. It does not begin explicitly. An addiction to a drug usually begins with *experimental use*. The experimental alcohol or other drug user lives in a society that encourages a certain degree of individual exploration. "Try this just once...then decide if you want more." Or, "I dare you to try this. Come on, show us what a man you are." Experimenting is a part of growing up. But sadly, many experimental users become *regular users*.

Experimental Use → Regular Use

Some regular users use drugs socially (social users), while others use drugs when they are alone (lone users). Both social use and lone use can get a person into *trouble-with* drugs.

Regular Use → Trouble-With Use
(social and/or lone use)

People who are in *trouble-with* drugs use them in the face of adverse effects to themselves (their health, their mind, their work), their families, their businesses, their neighborhoods or societies. It is easy to slip from regular use to trouble-with use because the early signs of trouble-with use are subtle and often go undetected. Someone who snorts a few lines of cocaine before leaving work, or who has a few drinks at a bar on the way home, is already driving "under the influence"—however slight that influence may seem—of drugs or alcohol. Driving home may be entirely possible. The point is that many users who are in a state of trouble-with use do not consider the risks that their use is posing to themselves or to others. They are not even aware of how easily they can slip from trouble-with use into *addictive use*.

Trouble-With Use → Addictive Use

Addictive use is enslavement. When the chemical memory calls, the craving for drugs wells up within the user. The user responds by using the drug, regardless of the pain, the costs, the risks, or the consequences.

The entire path from experimental to fully addictive use can be traced as follows:

Experimental → Regular → Trouble-With → Addictive

Fortunately, not every one who tries alcohol or drugs travels this tragic path. Some experimental users try a drink or drug once and then consider the experiment completed. But all too commonly, experimental users unwittingly slip into regular use. For example, many people are currently experimental or even regular users of alcohol or another drug. We are confidently telling ourselves, "It can't happen to me. I'm too much in control of my life to develop a drug problem. I'm just having a little fun." In reality, we are deluding ourselves. Case history after case history demonstrates that experimental use dramatically increases the probability of developing a fully addictive drug dependence. And using regularly increases the chances even more.

We have all experienced the tragedy of drug addiction. It happens to ourselves, or to our family members; to our friends, to our neighbors, to their children, to our fellow employees, to our bus drivers, our doctors, our nuclear power plant operators, or other members of our community. More often than not, the addiction problems of our society strike frighteningly close to home. We have all seen the addict—who lives among us, within us—who is us. We can no longer look away; the problem belongs to us all. And for many of us, the problem actually begins at home. Even if we are still in denial about our own explicit or implicit pattern addictions, we can help ourselves by understanding what it is that we share with explicit drug addiction.

3

Rethinking Recovery

In the era of the the war on drugs and the war on drug addiction, we became familiar with the standard jargon of addiction treatment. In that jargon, explicit addiction is called a *disease* and the time spent getting well is called a period of *recovery* from that disease. This jargon was borrowed from the lingo of medical care. According to this adaptation of language, once someone has been explicitly addicted, he or she will be a life-long *recovering addict*. This disease/recovery model has helped many thousands of people confront and then work through their explicit addiction problems. The concept of life-long recovery also helps friends and relatives appreciate the gravity of the problem and the continuing seriousness of addiction long after the addicted person has stopped drinking, drugging, or manifesting any other explicit addictive behavior.

But despite its utility, it is important that we recognize the philosophical limitations of the disease/recovery model and how these limitations affect the addicted person's ability to stop being addicted—or the sick person's ability to stop being ill.

First, while it is true that the disease/recovery model helps to remove some of the blame from our description of explicitly addicted persons, it does not really remove as much blame as we imagine it does. True, when addiction is viewed as a disease, it follows that it is not the addict's fault that he or she is addicted. In a society so eager to label explicit addicts as untouchables, as the dregs of society, the disease/recovery model provides some relief from the moral overtones of a blame-the-victim public outlook. Unfortunately, the model provides only some relief. A diseased person is still very often stigmatized and blamed for the disease in our society. This was as true of diseased lepers in ancient times as it is of persons with AIDS today.

The second philosophical limitation stemming from the disease/recovery model is that it allows the focus to remain on the individual rather than on society. The individual is viewed as having the unfortunate disease of addiction in an otherwise "well" society, rather than society or the world being viewed as being afflicted with the pervasive problem of detrimental pattern addiction. During the so-called "War on Drugs," media campaigns to "Call for Help" and "Just Say No" addressed the drug crisis as though drugs were only the problem of individuals. At least public funds were used to provide this information, which means that the public was involved in fighting this explicit addiction. But this is far short of what must be done to address the situation: all of society, all of the world, must focus a substantial portion of its attention, energy, and money on treating pattern addiction on a societal and global level. An effort on this level would require making transcendence-oriented treatment available to everyone, regardless of income, age, symptoms, addictions, or criminal record—essentially widespread across-the-board social programs with the enrollment of all citizens. It would also mean changing the emphasis of our public announcements from a "Just Say No" focus on the individual to a declaration that we are all part of the problem and are all therefore responsible for creating a solution.

A third limitation of the disease/recovery model is the view that the only positive change away from the "disease" is a state of life-long "recovery." There are no other positive options. There is no cure. The effect of this model is to limit the scope of behavior and self-definition available to someone who was once in trouble with an addiction. It limits people's concepts of themselves. They are told to think of themselves only as "recovering addicts." At best this is a half-truth. If people can be many things before becoming addicted, then they can be much more than simply "recovering addicts" after treatment. If they were fathers, mothers, lawyers, artists, or lovers before their addiction problems, they can continue to be these things after the problems have been addressed. The use of the term *recovery* is limiting in that:

> Recovery is the *only* positive mode of existence made available to a person who has been addicted.
> Recovery is the *only* life-challenge posed for the person who has been addicted.
> The nature of recovery, by its very name, is convalescence.
> Life-long convalescence imposes severe limits on people in that they are perpetually getting over a "bad thing that once happened."

Recovery thus invites a social stigma against "recovering addicts," in that they are labeled, for the rest of their lives, as "recovering addicts."

Recovery, in itself, is not necessarily *growth* , although many people grow psychologically and spiritually during recovery.

The fourth and last limitation of the disease/recovery model is that it limits our ability to think creatively about the nature of addiction. It prevents our addressing addiction from alternative perspectives. The disease model necessitates the use of the term *recovery*, which justifies the use of the disease model. This model prevents us from even considering the possibility that addiction is anything but individual sickness and its aftermath anything but getting well. We are ensnared in a philosophical conundrum, our minds and hearts trapped by the words we use.

Instead of viewing addiction as an illness that afflicts the individual, let's think of chemical dependence and of all pattern addiction as a challenge or struggle that some of our fellow humans are going through and making visible for all of us. *The addicted and afflicted among us are our pioneers, searching for a way out of individual, societal, and planetary stress.* They are alerting us to the chemicalization and mechanization of life on earth. They are manifesting our addictive materialism and addictive inadequacy so that we can examine it. They are warning us that our biotechnologies, our bodies and brains, can go wrong. They are exploring the frontiers of the human spirit and psyche, as others have explored uncharted continents on earth and still others will explore our solar system and even reach beyond to unknown regions of space. When the addicted among us find an answer to their personal dilemmas, no matter how large or small, they have made *discoveries* that bring enlightenment to us all. With this perspective in mind, the addicted individual, instead of being sentenced to a life of *recovery*, has the option of entering into a commitment to life-long *discovery*, what I call the *discovery model.*

The *discovery model* implies that postaddiction makes its actors the vanguard, even the leaders, in the realm of spiritual development. Persons who enter life-long discovery seek answers for themselves and for their fellow humans. In the transcendence of the crises of their addictions, these seekers are addressing the question, *"How can we as a society transcend the global crises being experienced by our species?"*

The modern world is loaded with crises. While social turmoil, hunger, disease, and war have been stressful throughout history, we have now entered a *global* era that allows us to feel the stress of crises in every country, city, and even family on earth. Even those individuals who have been relatively isolated from global stress are now being forced via television to cope with it on at least some level. There may or may not be some divine entity placing these crises in our paths out of a desire for us to grow. Maybe we generate them ourselves. Whatever the case may be, we can view them and the stress they cause as motivations for us as individuals and as a species to meet the challenges they present—and in the process of overcoming those challenges, to discover new ways of seeing and being.

Perhaps a new global spirituality will emerge once an understanding of the purpose of human suffering has been reached on this planet. In the meantime, countless individuals are enmeshed in what may, on some level, be a self-induced explicit addiction to drugs or food or money or work or sex. To some observers, explicit addiction, especially drug addiction, appears to be a "luxury problem" for people "who have nothing else to be troubled by." Nothing could be further from the truth. We have only to look across socioeconomic lines and into our own and other nations, large and small, rich and poor, to see that drug addiction is an insidious and, indeed, global reality. It affects the homeless on the streets of American cities, the hungry in Somalia or Biafra, and the peasants in the back-country hills of Burma every bit as much as the affluent of Beverly Hills. No matter who encounters the pain of addiction, it is the same—the great equalizer.

Addiction brings all people to their knees. Drug addiction acquaints everyone with the hazards of the larger war between the human soul and the forces that program and automate it. Drug-addicted people are at war with themselves, their struggle explicitly brutal, their carnage physical and spiritual, feeling themselves sucked into the black hole of enslavement to patterning every time they feel the craving—the inner screaming for their chemical switches. If they fight to control the urge to use drugs, they are at war with themselves. If they succumb to the urge and use them, they are at war with their environments, families, neighborhoods, work-places, worlds and themselves. This warring takes its toll on both the addicted persons and those around them. Death seems to be the only escape. Some die of overdoses; some kill themselves; some kill others while driving under the influence or while feeling paranoid and crazed from the drugs; some hurt their children so much that the children die inside or turn to drugs themselves in order to cope with the pain. But many addicts choose robotic lives over death. They simply allow their own hearts and souls to succumb to automatic, soulless programming. They are what we often call the "living dead," the soul dead. The light literally leaves their eyes, but they refuse to let their programming die. Transcendence is blocked. We are all involved in this anguish, this limbo. One way or another, we all feel its effects. Addiction is a world war, a spiritual struggle that alerts us to the global diminishment of human .freedom. We must thank drug addiction for teaching us this.

Addiction is a strange kind of enemy in that weapons best used against it are understanding, compassion, respect for human dignity, love and peace. Anyone who has worked with or lived with addicted individuals knows the need for these kinder, gentler weapons. In the field of drug addiction treatment, we have wandered the battlefields of the mind, body, and soul where this war between life and drugs—between transcendence and soul death—is raging. There are times when the automatic robotic side—the dark side—looks so very overpowering. Standard weapons do not work against it—only a sustained stream of light can drive the dark away.

Many persons who have been explicitly addicted have discovered that the key to moving past addiction is the development of a personal spirituality. Although their versions of spirituality differ, its importance is almost universally agreed upon. Sometimes the friends and family of a person who discovers life beyond addiction can see and feel the glow of this person's newfound spirituality. When they see this glow, they know that somehow, out of his or her suffering, the loved one who has been addicted is coming to terms with what it means to be alive, having somehow developed a reverence for life and discovered the great gift of being. Every crisis in such people's lives provides an opportunity for them to be "only human," to struggle and to overcome—to rise above, to see more, to travel to a new level of mastery, of being, of seeing—to *transcend.* These people have committed themselves to discovery, and their discoveries bring enlightenment to all of us.

It is time that we award explicitly addicted persons, and other people who are suffering or have suffered from illness, our respect, rather than simply setting them aside under the naive labels of *diseased* and *recovering from disease.* It is time that we understand the fundamental role that the person who has been pattern addicted can fill in our society. It is time that we rename "recovery," *discovery* and begin calling recovering pattern addicts *explorers* because that is what they really are.

Part II

Introduction to Practical Transcendence

One day I dreamed I was a butterfly.
—Chang-Tzu

4

Conditions for Transcendence

Whether or not it is physical, healthy death involves *transcendence*, one of the most special experiences one can have during one's lifetime. Transcendence is lifehealing. Many of our problems are encountered or created to provide us with the opportunity to transcend them, to heal our lives. As human beings we have a choice. We can either become so overwhelmed by our problems that we miss out on this amazing opportunity, or we can realize that addiction is a *potential-laden* situation.

Those who are addicted to a pattern (of drug use or eating or something more subtle, such as an emotional or energetic pattern) have a wonderful opportunity to experience transcendence—specifically to transcend addiction. Transcendence requires a new outlook on a situation. No matter how bleak and painful a situation may appear, it can be changed by being *reperceived* . This means that, before any changes can occur, you must be convinced of the fact that *you can turn things around!* You must believe in the possibility of transcendence. You must also understand the process, which must be studied and practiced continually. No matter what level of understanding you reach, there is always more to be learned. This and the following two chapters are a basic introduction to the process of transcendence. And while they deal somewhat more specifically with alcohol and drug addiction than with other addictions, the basic principles applied here can be applied to any kind of addictive behavior.

Remember, there is no such thing as a free lunch. Transcendence is hard work. In fact, there are the four basic conditions to full participation in the transcendence process: *commitment, attention, fortitude,* and *faith* in the process. These are interactive states of mind. Read slowly and carefully, and you will fully absorb the significance of each. Along with an explanation of each condition, exercises are provided as tools for personal development in each area. You will find a summary of these exercises, combined into an 8-week (56-day) program, at the end of this chapter.

COMMITMENT

The most basic condition for transcendence is the decision to make a commitment to the process. This does not just "happen." It is not something that you "stumble into." If it were, many people would be experiencing it "by chance" every day. The transcendence process described here requires a *total commitment,* a *heartful* tenacity and determination. It means putting everything on the line for change.

But just how do you develop commitment? It is easy to get all fired up about some words of encouragement that you read in a book. It's easy to say, "This is it. I'm going to change my life!" But excitement and commitment are not the same thing. Excitement is just a temporary high. Commitment is a process of practicing the same thing, every day, for a long, long period of time. The following exercises will help.

Decide to Be Committed

First of all, being committed requires making a conscious decision to be committed. It sounds simple, but many people find this initial decision difficult to make and hang on to. Making and keeping decisions takes practice.

Begin to experience the process of commitment by doing this exercise: Set aside six days out of your week, Monday through Saturday, to work on transcendence. Then take Sunday off as a little vacation for yourself. Or, if you like, take another day of the week off. Just make sure you choose the same day every week. Consistency will help you be firm about your decisions.

On the morning of the first day, make a conscious decision to be committed. Wake up and make the decision, and then really feel that decision for a day. Then, the next day, wake up and make a conscious decision not to be committed. Feel that lack of committment for the entire day. On the third day, repeat the first day. And on the fourth day, repeat the second day. Continue this on–off, committed–uncommitted exercise for two more days. This will total six days. You are alternating between deciding to be committed and deciding not to be committed. You will learn about commitment by experiencing the contrast between it and the absence of it. This exercise trains you to tell the difference. As you learn to do so, you will find that your committment gains clarity and strength. After this 6-day exercise, take your vacation day. (Refer to the schedule at the end of this chapter.)

When you are able to clearly make a decision to commit yourself to transcendence you will have overcome a major stumbling block. Many people who approach transcendence are interested in the profound personal, spiritual, emotional, and intellectual change that it entails, but are still somewhat afraid of that change. Because of this fear, they hesitate to truly commit to the process. Making this decision is the first step on the road.

Feel Committed

Commitment requires more than just a decision. A feeling must accompany that decision. Too often, people who want to change their lives have difficulty understanding what "commitment" means. This is because commitment must be felt, not simply talked about.

There is a difference between deciding to be committed and feeling committed. Decision rationally commands the intellect, the logical faculties of the mind, to carry out a specific set of actions or intentions. This is the necessary first step. The second step is feeling this commitment, which is more than employing one's logical faculties. We are talking about employing one's *psychological* faculties—getting one's feelings and emotions involved in the process.

Try this next exercise. Again, experiment by alternating days of commitment with days of noncommitment for six days. On the days that you are feeling committed, try to increase the level of feeling over the previous day's. Play act if you have to. Exaggerate your feelings, get "psyched up." Just make sure you get a good idea of what it might feel like to be really committed. If you continue this day-on, day-off process for six days, you will begin to get the sense that there is a difference between feeling committed and not feeling committed. By working on it, you can increase the degree of feeling in your commitment. The seventh day is, again, your day of rest.

Feel Committed on All Levels

Once you understand the difference between feeling committed and not feeling committed, it is important to look at commitment on various levels of your being. In this third step, you will add depth to the second step. Instead of simply feeling committed, you will learn to feel committed to specific areas of growth leading to transcendence.

There are many levels of being to which we must be committed if we are to experience transcendence. Among these are the intellectual level, the psychological or emotional level, the spiritual level, the physical level, and the economic or financial level. To be committed to transcendence is to be committed on all of these levels. To bring about purposeful transcedence, we must be committed so thoroughly, with so much feeling and on so many levels, that everything we think or do reflects that commitment. In other words, the whole person becomes committed. Every dollar spent is spent while feeling that commitment. Every hour spent is spent while feeling that commitment. Partial involvement in the process of commitment to transcendence is almost no involvement at all. The rules here apply to the whole mind, the whole self, and the whole heart. If you are to succeed, there can be no other, no higher, no competing allegiance. You must be loyal to your commitment to transcendence.

Practice feeling committed on an increasing number of levels for six days. On the first day of this six-day period, feel committed on one level, say the economic level. Any money you spend must be spent with your commitment in mind. On the second day, feel committed on the economic level and another level, say the physical. Everything you do with your body, you must do with your commitment in mind. And on each of the next four days add a new level of commitment and feel committed on all the levels you have selected up to that day. By the sixth day, you will have six levels upon which you are actualizing your commitment, that is, the economic, physical, nutritional, social, emotional, and time-management areas. Here are some examples of how to actualize your commitment on these various levels:

Economic—On this day, draw up a budget for the month; allow no expenditures on or in any way related to the object of your addiction. Apply the money you save toward some other cause—bill paying, therapy, health care, donations. Be highly conscious of your use of, and thoughts about, money on this day. Money represents economic energy. Learn about what money means to you.

Physical—On this day, carve out more time than you usually would to care for your body. Exercise, stretch, and bathe it well. Your body is the temple of your soul.

Nutritional—On this day, stop and pause before each bite of food that you take. Ask yourself if the food you are about to eat will nourish you. Thank the universe, or god as you know god, for nourishment.

Social—On this day, make each social contact reflect your commitment to transcendence. Say something about this exercise each time you speak to someone, even strangers. Be brave. Be open. Be honest.

Emotional—On this day, concentrate on each emotion that ripples through your soul. How much do you know about what you feel? How sensitive are you to what you feel? Find a way to connect each emotion to your sense of commitment.

Time management—On this day, plan your time out for the next month. During this first day of your new schedule, plan short breaks (even thirty seconds, if that's all you have time for) every hour to be certain you can feel your commitment. Time is a river. You are a passenger, an explorer in time. Chart the territory.

ATTENTION

Commitment is essential to transcedence. Attention is an equally important condition to the process of transcendence. There is no free lunch with this condition either. To achieve transcendence, one must *pay* attention. All too often, commitments are made and strongly felt, but a clear and continuing attention to the commitment is not maintained. Our minds wander at the slightest invitation. In order to learn transcendence, the student must pay tuition—in the form of attention. This is an exercise that will help you begin to pay attention. (Remember to refer to the schedule at the end of this chapter for guidance.)

Go Conscious

Open your eyes. Strive to see all there is to see. Go conscious as a way of staying out of your automatic habit mode. We are so much less conscious of the world around us than we can be. There is always room for greater observation. Most of us have never experienced higher states of perception. Some of us, however, have turned to drugs in order to achieve what we think of as a heightened state of perception. Drugs are viewed by some users as being a shortcut to these heightened states. The truth, however, is that drugs only produce an illusion of a heightened state, and a short lived one at that.

You can learn to achieve heightened states of perception without chemicals. You can actually learn to "go conscious." This means turning on your eyes, ears, sense of taste, of smell, of touch, even turning on your sixth sense—your intuition. Practice looking at everything around you. Spend one day deciding to see as much as possible. On the following day, decide not to see as much as possible. Spend the day after that seeing as much as possible again—you know the routine. Do it for six days. Learn that there is a difference. On the days when you are perceiving as much as possible, really go for it. Listen for sounds that you have never heard or never paid attention to before. Try to smell and taste things that go otherwise unnoticed. As you continue to alternate days, you will notice that you can continue to increase your level of sensory perception simply by deciding to do so. By concentrating on increasing your awareness, you will become conscious of the process.

Focus

Learning to focus is difficult. Most of us have not been taught to focus, that is, to truly concentrate. Do this exercise. Think of yourself using a precision camera, the lens of which you must focus manually. Use your hand to turn the ring on the lens until the image you are looking at through the camera comes into sharp focus. If it looks only somewhat sharp, you haven't gone far enough. Do not stop until the image is perfectly sharp. Only at this point are you in focus. Now take this experience and apply it to the way you perceive the world—to the way you see, hear, taste, smell, and feel. Your eyes are precision lenses. Your ears are ultrasensitive microphones. Your tongue is a sophisticated tasting machine. Your nose is a fine instrument for smelling the world. And your skin is a "lens" on all the things you touch and feel. Focus your "lenses." Continually sharpen your focus. Spend the next set of six days working on your focus. Focus a different sense each day, that is, day one: sight; day two: hearing; day three: taste; day four: smell; day five: touch; day six intuition. Rest on the seventh day.

Call Details Into Consciousness

After doing these exercises, you will find that you notice details more often and more clearly than ever before. You will find that you see shadows, reflections, nuances of color. You will begin to feel the texture of the foods you eat, the richness and variety of smells in the world, the feel of the wind on your skin.

As you notice more details, recognize that you are becoming more perceptive and strive to increase the quantity and clarity of the details that you experience. Whenever you find yourself with a free moment, sharpen your focus and look for details. Look hard for these details. Call them into your consciousness. They will not merely sit there, readily available for your examination. You will have to work hard to bring them there; you will have to say, "Come to me now, details."

When Your Mind Wanders, Refocus It

Your mind will wander. There will be times when you will not notice that it has wandered until an hour, half a day, a day, a week, a month, perhaps even a year has gone by. Don't let this discourage you. As soon as you notice that your mind has wandered, refocus it. Go back to thinking of yourself as a camera lens. Turn that ring; focus your mind.

Seek Intentional Awareness

Awareness of your surroundings does not happen by accident. You must choose to be aware. Awareness must be intentional, and this requires that you pay attention to what you are perceiving. Without intentional awareness, there can be no transcendence. So *pay attention.*

FORTITUDE

The greatest threat to a continuing commitment and attention to transcendence is a lack of fortitude. Fortitude is more than commitment and attention. When a person has fortitude, he or she can endure hardship, pain, and adversity with courage. Imagine the fortitude of the mountain climber who climbs through blizzards and below-freezing temperatures, who continues on the journey in the face of extreme hardship. With fortitude, the student of transcendence is unwavering, even in the face of problems and distractions. There may be countless obstacles to your progress: family fights, divorce, job loss, illness, discrimination, loneliness, and insecurity. These hardships call upon you to develop fortitude.

Learn to Recognize Your Fortitude

Decide again, as we have done with earlier exercises, to alternate days. On the first day you will decide to feel fortitude. On the second day you will decide not to feel fortitude. Continue in the normal alternating pattern. As you continue to alternate days, you will begin to notice the difference between feeling fortitude and not feeling it. Try to increase the feeling each day you decide to feel it. You will learn, as you have in other exercises, to detect two different types of experience. One is that you can feel your fortitude—you will be able to discern between the presence and absence of it. The other is that you can increase the *intensity* of the fortitude that you feel.

When a Problem Arises, Generate Fortitude

As you are working on the exercises described in this chapter, both unforeseen and predictable problems will confront you. They will interfere with your struggle for transcendence. You can however, use any obstacle or problem to generate strength and fortitude, as an opportunity to grow. You can turn it around. Any time a problem comes along, whether it is a ringing phone while you are trying to concentrate, news that your bank account is $5,000 overdrawn, or a sudden craving for drugs, use it as an opportunity to practice feeling fortitude, and as an opportunity to increase the intensity of that feeling with each new obstacle. Remember: use your problems to strengthen your fortitude.

FAITH

Faith is the ultimate condition for transcendence. Without it, there will be doubt in the process of transcendence and in oneself. Doubt can be hidden or obvious, subconscious or conscious. Whatever form it takes, it undermines the flow of energy into the transcendence process. The feeling of faith is subtle and may be difficult to experience in the beginning; but with practice and patience, faith grows stronger. Faith is a belief in the process of a transcendence. Faith is an optimism of the spirit, a hanging on to the positive view, no matter what argues against it. Survivors of shipwrecks and storms and other struggles often claim that they never lost faith. You too can learn not to lose faith by developing your ability to have faith.

Experience Faith

As you have done with other exercises, learn to experience faith by alternating days. On the morning of the first day, wake up and decide to experience faith all day. Overdramatize your faith. "Fake it till you make it" applies here. On the second day, decide to not experience faith. As you continue to alternate days, you will notice that you are learning about the difference between experiencing faith and not experiencing faith. Through this difference you will begin to learn what it means to have faith.

Strengthen Faith

The development of faith is probably one of the most important components in the entire process of learning transcendence. On each day that you decide to experience faith, decide to experience more of it than you did the previous day. You will learn, as you have with the other exercises, that once you are able to recognize a feeling, you can learn to develop and strengthen that feeling.

The stronger your faith, the more power and energy you will be able to direct into the process of transcendence. Your faith will grow from a trickle into a rushing river of energy, flowing from you to you, from the world around you to you, and from you into the world around you. Commit yourself to strengthening your faith. You will feel the abundant rewards.

Sustain Faith

Once you have learned to recognize faith and your ability to strengthen it, you must work to sustain it. When you feel faith, say to yourself, "Oh, this is what faith feels like, and this is what it feels like to decide to have it and then to actually follow through on strengthening my faith. And this is what it feels like to strengthen faith. Now that I've experienced it, I'm not going to let it go. I'm going to sustain this feeling of strong faith." Learning to sustain faith is like learning to ride a bicycle. At first it will be difficult to keep your balance. You will be able to sustain your faith for a little while and then you may begin to waver and lose your balance. But if you keep trying, you will eventually find that you can strengthen your faith and hang on to it. And once you have truly learned to sustain your faith, you will not unlearn it. Try sustaining your faith for six consecutive days.

CONDITIONS FOR TRANSCENDENCE

That's it! These conditions—commitment, attention, fortitude and faith—must be continuously developed. There is always room to grow. Fix these conditions in your mind and continuously repeat the above exercises and address the above considerations until you develop your own exercises for strengthening your commitment, attention, fortitude, and faith in the transcendence process. Life will present you with tests of your progress. You can count on this.

Remember the conditions:

Conditions for Transcendence

Commitment

Decide to be committed.
Feel committed.
Feel committed on all levels.

Attention

Go conscious.
Focus.
Call details into consciousness.
When your mind wanders, refocus it.
Seek intentional awareness.

Fortitude

Learn to recognize your fortitude
When a problem arises, generate fortitude.

Faith

Experience faith.
Strengthen faith.
Sustain faith.

Use the following 8-week schedule your first time through these exercises to see how they build on each other. Repeat this schedule, as is or in an amended form, at least ten times. As you grow used to meeting the conditions for transcendence write yourself a schedule for practicing two or three conditions at the same time.

SCHEDULE FOR DEVELOPING REQUISITES FOR TRANSCENDENCE

Day #	Commitment	Attention	Fortitude	Faith	Your Notes
1	decide to be committed				
2	decide nothing				
3	decide to be committed				

Day #		Commitment	Attention	Fortitude	Faith	Your Notes
4		decide nothing				
5		decide to be committed				
6		decide nothing				
7		day of rest				
8	(1)	decide to be committed and *feel* committed				
9	(2)	do not feel committed				
10	(3)	feel more committed				
11	(4)	do not feel committed				
12	(5)	feel even more committed				
13	(6)	do not feel committed				
14	(7)	day of rest				
15	(1)	feel committed on a new level (i.e., economic)				
16	(2)	feel committed on a new level (i.e., physical)				
17	(3)	feel committed on a new level (i.e., nutritional)				
18	(4)	feel committed on a new level (i.e., social)				
19	(5)	feel committed on a new level (i.e., emotional)				
20	(6)	feel committed on a new level (i.e., time management)				
21	(7)	day of rest				

Day #	Commitment	Attention	Fortitude	Faith	Your Notes
22	(1)	go conscious: decide to see as much as possible			
23	(2)	do not try to see as much as possible			
24	(3)	decide to see as much as possible			
25	(4)	do not try to see as much as possible			
26	(5)	decide to see as much as possible			
27	(6)	do not try to see as much as possible			
28	(7)	day of rest			
29	(1)	sharpen your focus: decide to see as much as possible and increase your level of sensory perception in one area (i.e., sight)			
30	(2)	sharpen your focus: decide to see as much as possible and increase your level of sensory perception in one area (i.e., hearing)			
31	(3)	sharpen your focus: decide to see as much as possible and increase your level of sensory perception in one area (i.e., taste)			
32	(4)	sharpen your focus: decide to see as much as possible and increase your level of sensory perception in one area (i.e., smell)			

Day #	Commitment	Attention	Fortitude	Faith	Your Notes
33 (5)		sharpen your focus: decide to see as much as possible and increase your level of sensory perception in one area (i.e., touch)			
34 (6)		sharpen your focus: decide to see as much as possible and increase your level of sensory perception in one area (i.e., intuition) — sharpen your focus and call details into your consciousness. When your mind wanders, refocus it.			
35 (7)		day of rest			
36 (1)			decide to feel fortitude. When a problem arises generate fortitude.		
37 (2)			decide not to feel fortitude		
38 (3)			decide to feel fortitude		
39 (4)			decide not to feel fortitude		
40 (5)			decide to feel fortitude		
41 (6)			decide not to feel fortitude		
42 (7)			day of rest		
43 (1)				experience faith all day	
44 (2)				decide not to experience faith	

Day #	Commitment	Attention	Fortitude	Faith	Your Notes
45 (3)				experience faith <u>and</u> <u>strengthen</u> <u>it</u>	
46 (4)				decide not to experience faith	
47 (5)				experience faith and strengthen it	
48 (6)				decide not to experience faith	
49 (7)				day of rest	
50 (1)				experience faith and sustain faith	
51 (2)				sustain faith	
52 (3)				sustain faith	
53 (4)				sustain faith	
54 (5)				sustain faith	
55 (6)				sustain faith	
56 (7)				day of rest	

NEXT: repeat this schedule or write your own schedule combining exercises to allow you to practice various conditions for transcendence at the same time.

5

Phases of Transcendence

Transcendence is a continuous process through which an individual achieves elevation to a higher spiritual plane. Transcendence is composed of four profound phases, each of which is necessary for the process, and each of which is enhanced by the conditions described in the previous chapter. The phases of transcendence are:

    Phase 1:—Struggle
    Phase 2:—Paradox
    Phase 3:—Insight
    Phase 4:—Spiritual Elevation

PHASE CHARACTERISTICS

Each phase has its own special characteristics. I have included diagrams of these phases. As you examine each diagram, try to think of your life in terms of it. Make the diagrams part of your own mental imagery. Thinking in pictures often helps to learn on a deeper level.

Phase 1: Struggle

Every day we struggle—with other people, with family relationships, with work relationships, with ourselves, with morality, and maybe also with our cravings for drugs, with balancing our checkbooks, with heavy traffic, with our health, with our tempers, with our moods, with living up to what we think we or others would like to see us live up to. We often struggle without recognizing or seeing beyond it, becoming so deeply caught up that it becomes impossible to step back and say, "Oh, I am struggling. This must be the first phase of transcendence." But it is just this observation that will set us on the path to transcendence. When we are struggling we must take the time to tell ourselves that we *are* —and that that is good, because it is the first phase of transcendence.

Study Figure 5.1. This pattern illustrates ups and downs, pushes and pulls, and highs and lows so typical of the struggling phase. During a true struggle, there must be low points in order for there to be high points— both extremes are integral to it.

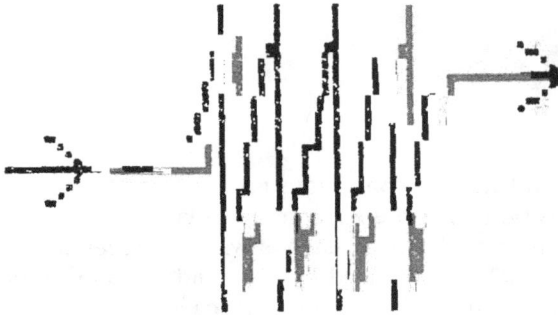

Figure 5.1.   **PHASE 1: Struggle**

Phase 2: Paradox

Paradox is a fantastic experience. It can be painful. It can be frightening. It can be deadly. It can produce a zombielike effect in those who experience it. Paradox is the experience of being in a situation from which there seems to be no escape, no resolution. The person in paradox feels trapped. Sometimes parents offer children paradoxes in the form of a double bind, something like this:

"Which coat do you like?" a parent may ask a child. "The red coat or the blue one?" If when the child says, "The red coat," the parent says, "That's not a good choice, you should like the blue one." And when the child says, "The blue one," the parent says, "Well, the red one is much better." When this happens, the child is experiencing a double bind. In this case there is nothing the child can do that would be the right thing to elicit a positive response from the parent. The child is bound by an unpleasant consequence no matter which choice he or she makes. There is no escape. The situation holds, or so it would seem, no real choices. In living life both children and adults create double bind situations for themselves with or without the help of other people.

One double bind that many people find themselves in these days is chemical dependence. The individual takes a drug to escape a painful, stressful, or boring situation. But the situation from which the person is trying to escape becomes even more painful, stressful, or boring when the person returns to it, as is inevitable upon coming down from the trip. While no escape is no escape, the drug escape is also no escape.

Paradoxes like this are extremely stressful and often painful. But faith in the transcendence process shows us that paradox serves a purpose. Without the tension, the feeling of being trapped in an unwinnable situation, there is no impetus for moving on. The tension created by your paradoxes, when used well, can generate enough energy for you to break out of them. Without the pain of paradox, we cannot experience the release—the jump or shift in perception that is produced by breaking out of the double bind.

Paradox is illustrated in Figure 5.2. Study it for a few minutes. It evokes the "stand off" or "holding pattern" in which people who need to grow and experience transcendence get caught or trap themselves. The only way out of this holding pattern is to grow past it, break out of it and move on, increase your perception so that you can see beyond the limits of the double bind that holds you there. The two arrows ending up against each other and going nowhere represent the forces that hold an addicted person in his or her trap. One force is the powerful tendency to stay stuck or addicted, to use drugs to avoid stress and pain. The other is the stressful and painful effect of drug use that seeks to avoid stress and pain. This deadlock can hold you in its grip indefinitely. Or, if you choose the way of transcendence, it can provide a take-off point into another level of being. When the paradox of addiction explodes, energy is released and this energy can bring insight. Whatever your addiction, you can harness the energy in its paradox and then move into transcendence. To do so, you must become highly alert to the tensions you feel and to your implicit pattern addictions which generate them.

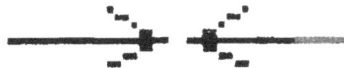

Figure 5.2. **PHASE 2: Paradox**

Phase 3: Insight

Insight is a profound experience. But it often comes in small packages. Sometimes we experience it without even realizing it. You may be driving along and suddenly grasp something about a problem that has been bothering you. Or you may be working—perhaps on a scientific or a construction project—and suddenly figure out an unexpected solution. All at once a new idea comes into your mind. You suddenly discover a new way of looking at a problem. This is an insight.

Insight is illustrated graphically in Figure 5.3. Look at the figure for a while. It suggests the glimpse, or perception, of another way of seeing the world and of being in the world. The highest point in this diagram is this flash of realization. It represents a peek (and a peak) into a higher level of experience. Now notice that the line falls back or almost back, to its original level. This is because insight is a temporary jump in perception. It does not automatically bring growth. In order to grow, insight must be recognized and sustained. When it is, spiritual elevation becomes a reality.

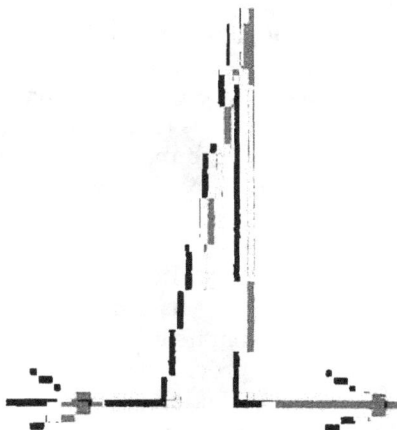

Figure 5.3.   PHASE 3: Insight

Phase 4: Spiritual Elevation

Spiritual elevation is illustrated in Figure 5.4. Gaze at it. What does this diagram symbolize to you? This pattern signifies a jump in perception. This jump is actually an insight that is *sustained*. The self, the soul, the spirit, rises to a new level of being and maintains it. This "holding on" is the experience of sustained insight. Without it, the insight is usually brief, and the people experiencing the insight return to or close to their original ways of seeing the world, as was seen in Figure 5.3. Spiritual elevation

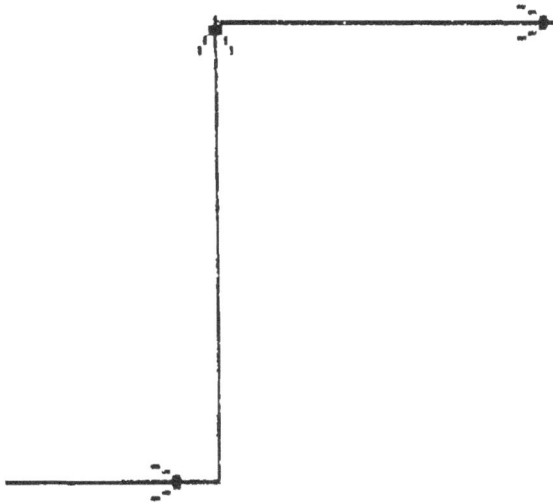

Figure 5.4. PHASE 4: Spiritual Elevation

differs from insight in that there is no going back to one's previous perceptions.

From the new level of being achieved by spiritual elevation, each of the phases of transcendence may have to be repeated in order to reach further spiritual elevation. One can always discover new struggles, paradoxes, and insights to generate further spiritual growth.

This exciting and adventurous process of transcendence is suggested in Figure 5.5. It shows the four phases of transcendence linked together. The cycle of phases is repeatable, as in Figure 5.7. Contemplate these diagrams for a while.

Be certain that you understand that each phase may take barely a few seconds or last for years. Some people struggle all their lives. Others live in a perpetual stage of paradox. Some rotate between struggle and paradox, as Figure 5.6 demonstrates. Perhaps these people reach spiritual elevation at death. Some people have insights but do not recognize or sustain them, and thus continuously return to the same paradox that produced these insights.

Each of us follows his or her own life pattern. However, no one's pattern is written in stone. If we were taught as children to recognize these phases of transcendence, then, as adults, it would be much easier for us to see where we are in the process and to take conscious control of

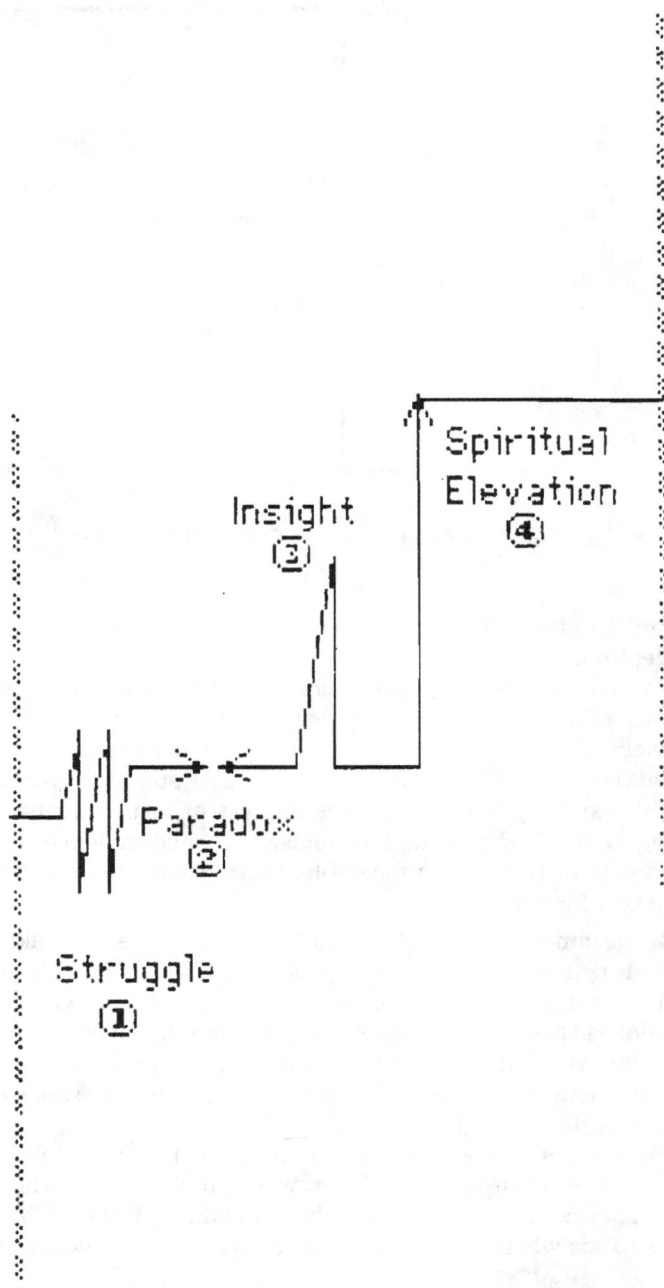

Insight ③

Spiritual Elevation ④

Paradox ②

Struggle ①

Figure 5.5.   The Four Phases of Transcendence

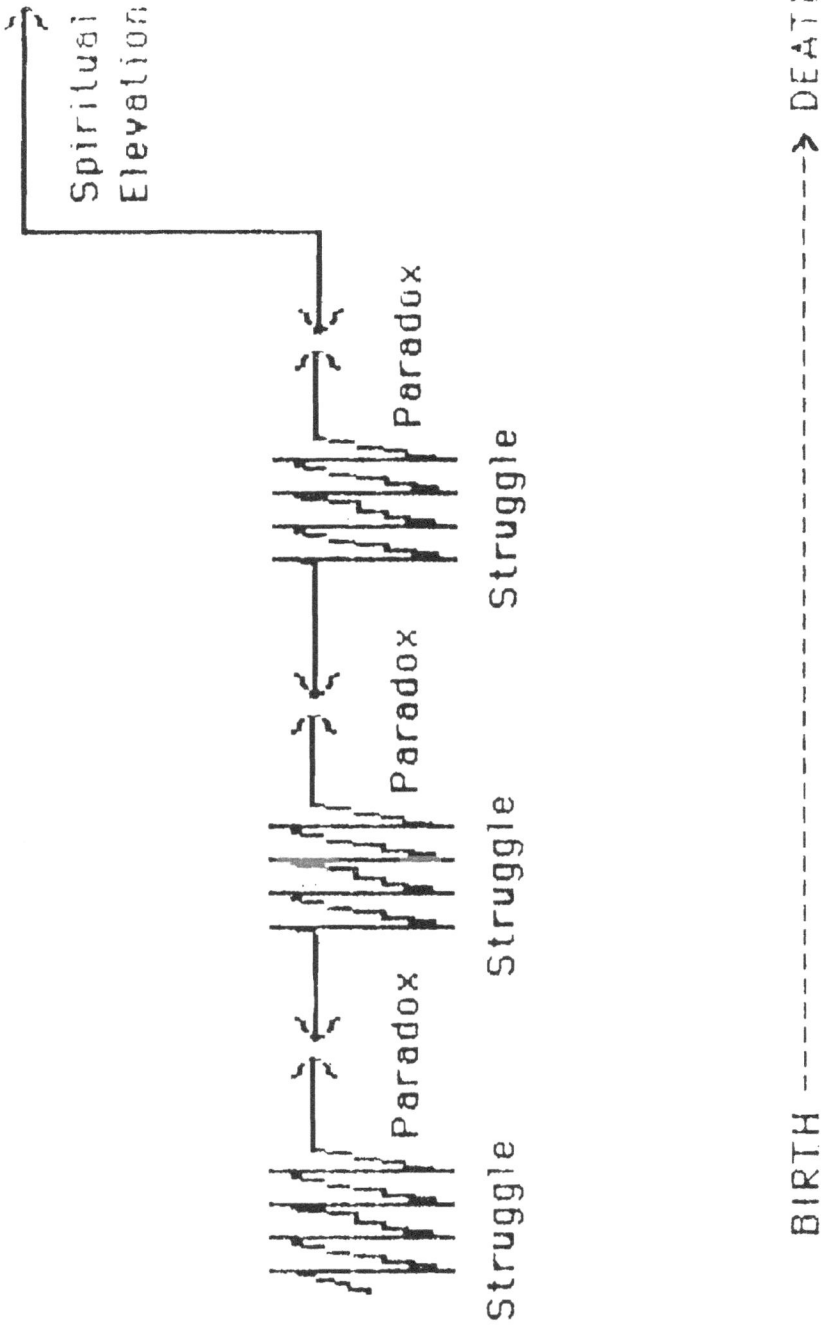

Figure 5.6.   Rotation Between Struggle & Paradox

47

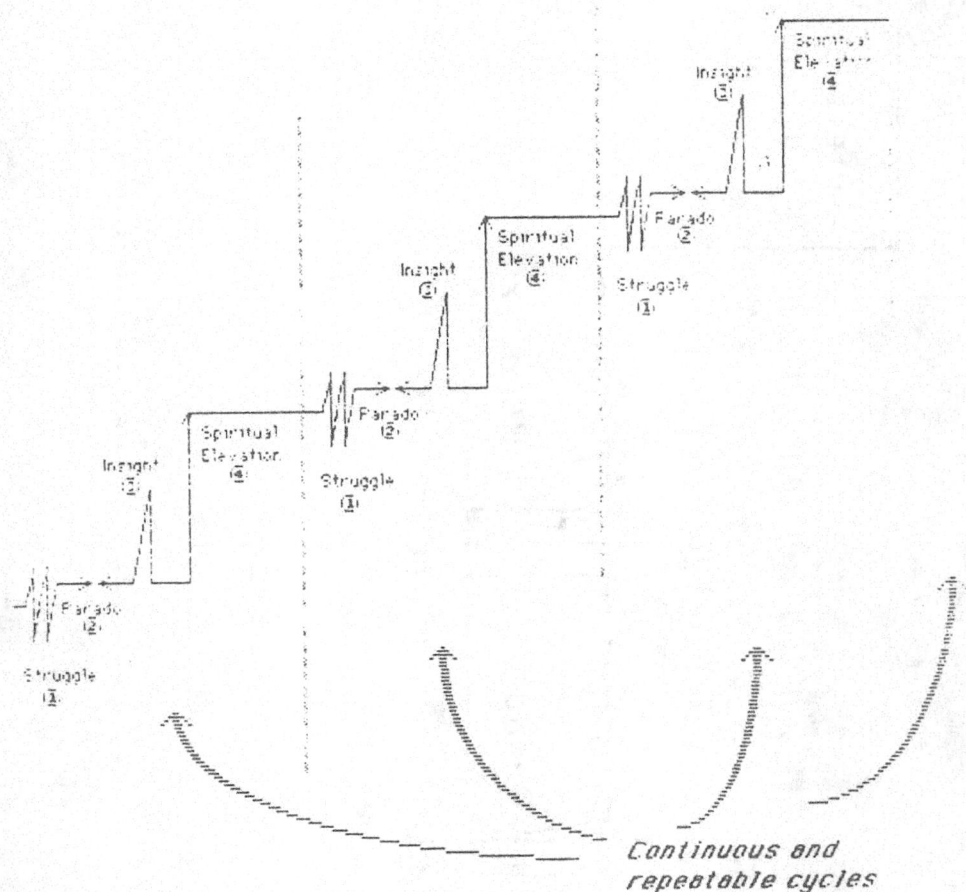

Figure 5.7. The Process of Transcendence

it. But no matter how old we are, we can always learn to harness the energy produced in each phase to move on to the next phase. We can learn to see our struggles as fertile ground for astounding growth. We can learn to appreciate paradox, recognize insight, and strive for spiritual elevation. If you keep trying to see this pattern in your life you will eventually understand that you are already on the path of transcendence. The gift of life will then make itself very clear to you. Your struggles are important stepping stones. Respect your struggles.

6

Seven Basic Ideas for Transcending Addiction

W e have spent the last two chapters analyzing the concept of transcendence—what it is, and what it takes to achieve it. The concept can be applied to any obstacle or difficulty we encounter, whether it be emotional, financial, physical, or another type of problem. Remember, even chronic and serious illnesses have a pattern-addiction component. Addiction to a pattern, any pattern, is the specific problem being addressed in this book, but the transcendence I describe is infinitely transferable. Addiction, whether it be to a drug or to a relationship, or to something else, offers everyone lessons in transcendence. Let's take the time to consider seven basic ideas about transcendence as it relates to addiction.

SEVEN BASIC IDEAS

Idea One

Addiction to a pattern is a powerful bondage that can only be broken by something more powerful. One must accept this as a fact and appreciate the size and seriousness of the task of breaking pattern addiction.

Idea Two

Pattern addiction can be very subtle and difficult to recognize. Therefore some individuals either present themselves, or are presented, with the challenge of an explicit addiction so that they may recognize how addicted to patterning we all are. They then undergo the struggle to break out of their most explicit addictive patterns and, in the process of that struggle, experience growth. Some people have found the recognition of addiction to be their primary opportunity for growth. Drug, alcohol, food and gambling addictions are some of the easiest patterns to spot and thus offer some of the most accessible opportunity to practice transcendence and to grow. Yet we all are pattern addicts.

Idea Three

The ultimate form of learning is transcendence, a process composed of four phases: struggle, paradox, insight, and spiritual elevation. This pattern is a repetative, never-ending process. Your entire experience of living is transformed the moment you identify the phase of the process you are currently experiencing.

Idea Four

One way to promote insight, spiritual elevation, and thus transcendence is through the pain, struggle, and paradox of addiction. There are many ways to encourage transcendence; addicted individuals have *selected* the vehicle of addiction to reach their goal of transcendence and discovery. Emotionally troubled and physically ill individuals have also selected the vehicle of pattern addiction as an opportunity to learn to transcend; however, this is not as obvious to people who do not have one of the more explicit addictions, such as those to alcohol or other drugs.

Idea Five

Remember that the transcendence we are describing is a process that gains power as it progresses. Progressive transcendence can overcome addiction and then move beyond. *There is no end point to this process.*

Idea Six

One must *work* to maintain the insights and spiritual elevations gained in the process of transcendence.

Idea Seven

With every full cycle of transcendence comes an entirely new way of seeing the self and the world. Be ready and open to total change and new life.

Only total change and an ongoing commitment to transcendence will heal the wounds to the soul that are caused by addiction. And only massive transcendence will heal the world. As the human species becomes more aware of its ability to consciously choose to transcend the trap of patterning in the physical world, it will ascend to the realm of the spirit. Biological death is not the only means of such ascendence.

It is essential that every one of us commit to spiritual development. Both personal and planetary pressures are calling us into action. Lifestyle change, when incorporated with the steps to spiritual change or transcendence presented in the previous chapters, is exciting and challenging. This type of change is no small event in a person's life. Read on. There is much to explore in the area of lifestyle change, for good life management must accompany your spiritual development.

Part III

Transcending Addiction to One's Programming

Life is either a great adventure or nothing.
—Helen Keller

7

Lifestyle Surgery: Breaking Addiction

The counterpart of spiritual development is life management. While spiritual development deals with the immaterial, abstract, esoteric part of human existence, life management deals with the material, practical, down-to-earth aspects of being a person. To conquer addiction, spiritual development and life management must work hand in hand. The qualitative juxtaposition of these two areas of personal development creates both a growth-producing tension and a nourishing balance.

The reason that life management skills are so important is that many addicted and otherwise troubled individuals have a difficult time with the job of just being a person. Their personal lifestyles are often disorganized, disrupted, and discombobulated. Whether this disorganization causes addictions, or whether the more explicit addictions cause this disorganization, is irrelevant. What is important is to realize that there is some relationship or connection between these factors. Poor life management skills make an addicted person much more vulnerable to addiction. When life is disorganized, it is much easier for people to fall prey to the whims of the powerful addictive programming they have stored in their bodies.

THE IMPORTANCE OF MANAGEMENT

Consider the legal concept "The dead hand reaches out." This describes the ability of someone who writes a will to influence the distribution of his or her estate long after he or she has died. This "dead hand" reaches out into the realm of the living—from the past into the present.

Addiction acts in a similar way. Let's look at how the dead hand of addiction reaches out. Addicted people have repeated their addictive behaviors, including countless actual physical motions and gestures, so many times that eventually they simply "go through the motions" of their addictions automatically. Many people who try to break even simple habits, such as fingernail biting, find that they perform their habits without thinking about them. Whether a relatively simple habit like nail biting, or a more intense habit, such as an addiction to drugs, the behavior has been repeated so often that it has worn a memory pathway through the brain and nervous system. This memory pathway can be thought of as a deep ravine into which spill connected sensations, memories, and gestures. For example, a man who has spent ten years biting his fingernails while watching television may find that, each time he sits down to watch television, his hand automatically ends up at his mouth. If he does not pay very close attention to what he is doing, he will unconsciously begin biting his nails. Likewise, a man who has been drinking or using drugs at social gatherings for fifteen years may find that, every time he is in the company of three or more people, he craves his old drink or drug. In this situation it is likely that, if he breaks down and "has just one," he will slip easily into having another and another, without paying any attention to what he is doing.

Memories of addicted individuals are like the will writer's dead hand—they reach out into the land of the living. They reach into the present from the past. They can reach out long after the addiction has been, or seems to have been, put to rest. The only way for a person who has been addicted to gain control over the powerful programing he has stored in memory—burned into brain cells—is *to manage his life very carefully.* Only by paying careful attention to every aspect of his life can he control the automatic behavior that will seek to control him. To win out over the insidious, intrusive, and seemingly omnipotent dead hand that addiction creates, concentration on life management skills is absolutely essential.

When addicted people gain an understanding of just how effective a job they have done, of how well they have programed their addictive behaviors into their mental circuitries, they can feel very discouraged, frightened, and overwhelmed. If you are addicted to something, you may be feeling this way right now.

"I'll never change. This pattern is in me too deeply. It controls me. I can't control it." These fears will continue to pop up until you learn self-confidence and self-control through life management. You need life management tools for change, to conquer your impulses. With these tools, profound change can become a reality in your life.

Most of us have not really experienced how good a healthy approach to organization feels. We either compulsively overorganize or we weakly underorganize. Either extreme fails to address basic management issues and fails to integrate all of the levels of life management into a stable, healthy, and energetic package.

Once some experience and skill in life management has been gained, a person who is trying to overcome a behavioral hurdle will increase confidence. And increased self-confidence brings *hope*, which makes personal change possible, no matter how large the obstacles to change seem to be. In developing management skills, addicted individuals learn that they actually can override their deeply entrenched programming.

OVERCOMING PROGRAMMING

A man who has taken twenty swallows of wine (approximately two glasses, depending on the size of the swallows) a day for five years— 36,500 swallows—has lifted a glass to his mouth and swallowed alcohol at least 36,500 times. The physical gesture of bringing the glass to one's mouth, the act of drinking and swallowing, and the psychological experience of tasting and absorbing alcohol into the system, are remembered along with the places, times, people, physical feelings, and emotions that have been repeatedly associated with those gestures. By sipping alcohol over and over again, this person has programmed himself to connect the gestures of drinking and swallowing with the experience of absorbing alcohol into his system and with all those events, places, people, and feelings. Any part of this memory configuration, a particular gesture or feeling or place or person, may call back the entire memory and reactivate the programing. That "little addict person" who lives in his nervous system and brain cells wakes up again. Because so many levels of existence are tied into the addicted person's memory configuration, an experience or action on any level of existence can trigger addictive behavior on any other level. This is why an individual seeking to change his or her programming must pay careful attention to all levels of his or her existence.

Addictive behavior is automatic and subconscious. To override an automatic, subconscious behavior, one must become highly *conscious* of that behavior. The breaking of an addictive behavior cannot be left to chance. *Pay attention*, a lot of attention.

DOING SOMETHING NEW

Addictive behavior takes many forms. Every person who is addicted has at least one, if not many, very personal addictive patterns. Nevertheless, it is possible to generalize these patterns and to construct a simple three-point addiction cycle that will give us insight into the nature of all addictive patterns. *(See Figure 7.1.)*

BREAK THE ADDICTIVE CYCLE

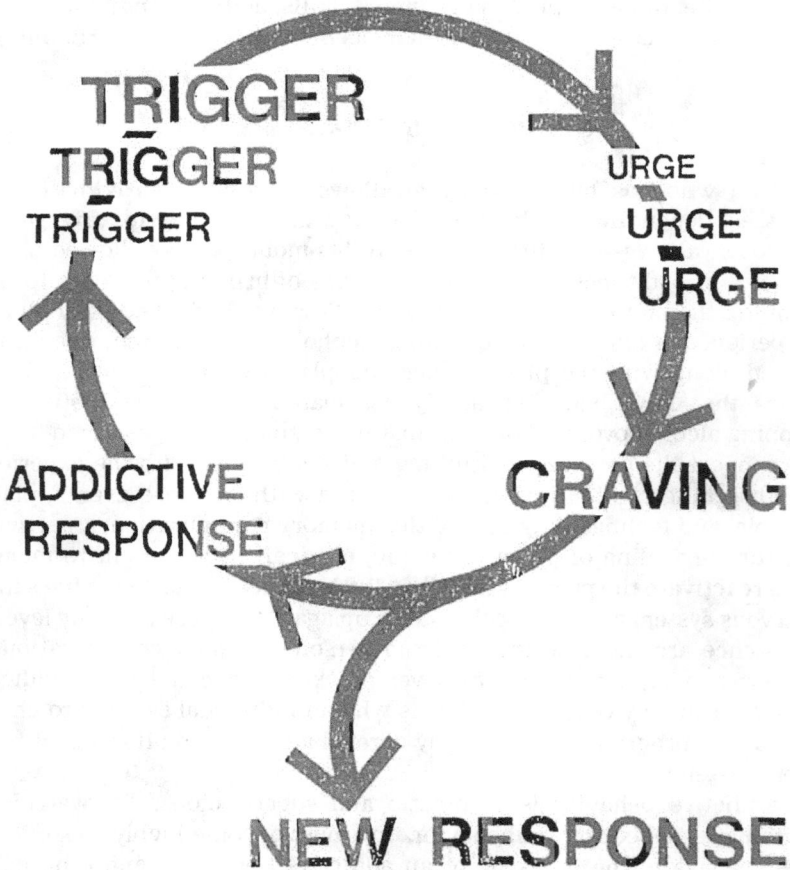

TRIGGER
TRIGGER
TRIGGER

URGE
URGE
URGE

ADDICTIVE RESPONSE

CRAVING

NEW RESPONSE

Figure 7.1. Break The Cycle Chart

The cycle usually begins when a deeply ingrained *trigger* causes the addicted person to feel the *urge* or craving to use the substance or to perform the action part of the pattern to which he or she is addicted. If the cycle continues, as it usually does, the addicted person actually responds to the urge with his or her *addictive response.* You will find these cycle points in Figure 7.1.

Breaking addiction requires breaking the cycle at one or more of these points. At cycle point one, triggers can be identified. Once they are identified, triggers can be eliminated, altered, or perceptions of them changed—depending on the nature of the trigger. When this has been successfully done, the cycle will be broken. When the addicted person experiences one of the triggers, it will no longer set off further movement through the cycle.

The cycle can also be broken at point two. Here urges (or cravings) can be identified, controlled, and lived through, provided that close attention is paid to the nature and course of one's urges. A break in the cycle at this point means that the urges will cease to lead to addictive responses. Finally, at cycle point three, addictive responses can be replaced with other, new responses. When the old addictive cycle is broken, something new happens.

One of the greatest obstacles in overcoming addiction to any pattern is *overcoming the resistance to change.* All too often the addicted individual is reluctant to change because change necessitates moving into the unknown, in other words, *doing something new.* This is why the process of breaking the addiction cycle must incorporate some highly methodical elements. There is no secret or magic recipe for transcending addiction. As we know, it takes a great deal of commitment and hard work. But this commitment must be backed up by a willingness to undergo radical change. We must be willing to perform *lifestyle surgery* on ourselves, to make whatever changes are necessary to break the addictive cycle. At the end of this chapter, you will find is an outline for effective lifestyle surgery.

Lifestyle surgery is not a magic process requiring little or no effort. Breaking addiction takes a difficult, and sometimes very mundane, daily injection of discipline. The first step is to identify and map the triggers in your life that lead to your addictive responses. You will receive direction in this area in Chapters 8 and 9. Once you begin this process, you can apply the life management plan that I detail in Chapter 10.

Lifestyle Surgery:
An Outline for Cutting Into the Habit Pattern

Triggers: Know Your Triggers

Identify your triggers.

Continue to identify more of your triggers.

Look for connections between your triggers. Find places where you can change the patterns by breaking the connections.

With each trigger you identify:
- eliminate it *or*
- stay away from it *or*
- change it *or*
- change your perception of it *or*
- learn to live with it.

Urges: Live Through Your Urges and Cravings

Recognize an urge.

Know that you can experience an urge without responding to it with your addictive behavior.

Understand that every urge will come to an end. You *can* live *through* an urge.

Responses: Change Your Responses

Replace your addictive responses with new responses.

Continuously improve your life management skills.

Stay in touch with your feelings.

Communicate your experiences.

Know when you need help and get it.

Aim for ongoing personal growth and discovery.

Do something new.

8

A Dictionary of Triggers

$\mathbf{O}$ne of the most important steps in breaking an addictive pattern is to identify the *triggers* that have been deeply embedded in that pattern. By recognizing these triggers, pattern-addicted people can take concrete steps to either change their triggers or change their responses to those triggers.

Remember that a trigger is anything that the addicted individual thinks of as being or responds to as a trigger. You already know this on some deep level if your are addicted: triggers are all in your mind. Sure, there are real things in the world that affect you, but your *reaction to anything and everything is generated by you* ! A trigger can be anything that sets off your desire to use alcohol or drugs. A trigger can be any object, experience, event, relationship, person, predicament, idea, or impulse that sets off or magnifies a chain of events. As a pattern-addicted individual, you are continually surrounded by, and experiencing, a variety of emotional, practical, social, psychological, physical, and chemical triggers. You must identify—become conscious of—as many of your triggers as you can in order to control their influence on you. Bring important data about yourself out of your subconscious and into your consciousness. This will help you pay better attention to yourself.

This chapter provides examples of over thirty triggers and categorizes them into ten problem areas. It will help you make your own list of your own triggers. The triggers listed here are, in the main, triggers of explicit addictive behaviors such as cyclical drug use, spending, and eating. As you read through this chapter, go ahead and write down your own list of triggers. Copy the triggers listed here if you feel that they pertain to you. Add anything else that comes to your mind—that the lists trigger in your mind—even ideas that may represent more implicit triggers. Write down *everything* that comes to mind, even if you do not have a category for it, even if you cannot explain it. You are brainstorming now.

PROBLEM AREA ONE: *PRACTICAL TRIGGERS*

Practical triggers are those which make it easy, that is, "practical," to obtain and to use the objects, or to do the behavior, of your addiction. Among those practical triggers most commonly listed by addicted individuals are:

Availability of Money With Which to Purchase the Objects of One's Addiction: such as cash on hand, too much money, too much credit, a bank card that makes it possible to get cash when the bank is closed.

Affordability: the object of one's addiction is affordable—often in large quantities—to the addicted individual.

Paybacks and Favors: gifts or returns of favors (i.e., in the form of alcohol or drugs given to the drug-addicted person).

Proximity: the source of the object of one's addiction (such as alcohol or drugs) is located nearby.

Invisibility: energy pattern problems are frequently invisible to untrained observers, and, therefore, the mere invisibility of problem energy patterns makes it practical to continue to have them.

PROBLEM AREA TWO: *TEMPORAL TRIGGERS*

Temporal triggers are all those time-related factors that influence or are connected with addictive behavior. Time periods of activity or inactivity and particular times of the day, week, month or year may have meaning to an addicted person. Common temporal triggers are:

Free Time: having enough time to reinforce and respond to one's programming often brings that programming out. (This is one of the most common triggers.)

Lack of Time: time-shortage conditions can also bring out one's automatic behaviors, because when there is no time to think about what one is doing, one just does whatever is programmed in—runs on automatic.

Particular Times of the Day: certain times such as family times, meal times, the "happy hour," the time right before or right after a workday begins or ends.

Particular Times of the Month: for example, many women report anticipated and actual premenstrual stress as a trigger, and some men also report monthly behavioral cycles; the full moon is listed by some as a trigger time. Hormonal and even gravitational changes are cyclical, and neurological patterning can be built around them.

Particular Times of the Year: these include winter months, the first hot spell, etc. Seasonal changes can, over the years, bring out automatic emotional and behavioral shifts.

All the Time: even the passage of time triggers some addictive behavior, and getting time to pass is the goal of a great deal of addictive behavior.

PROBLEM AREA THREE:
ENVIRONMENTAL TRIGGERS

Addicted persons are reminded of their previous addictive behaviors, and of other triggers, by their environments. Environmental triggers clearly bring out explicit addictive behaviors, but they also trigger implicit pattern cycles. For example, we all have seen how family members tend to fall into childhood roles at holiday get togethers in elder parents' homes. While this list focuses on triggers of explicit addictive cycles, the transfer to the implicit is easily made. Typical environmental triggers include:

Particular Cities
Specific Street Corners
Bars and Restaurants
Particular Houses
A Room in a House: the bathroom, the kitchen, the room with a bar, and any room associated with the habitual behavior.

Furniture and Appliances: mirrors, refrigerators, dresser drawers where "stashes" (i.e., secret stores of alcohol or drugs or food or money) are kept, and often furniture and appliances can be triggers.

Outdoor Environments: beaches, forests, sports stadiums.

Vehicles: i.e., cars and planes on long trips.

Particular Objects: the paraphernalia associated with the preparation for using an addictive substance, and any other objects identified with other triggers. OBJECT TRIGGERS can easily become a separate category.

PROBLEM AREA FOUR:
MEDIA TRIGGERS

The media are loaded with triggers for the pattern-addicted individual. Again, familiarity and association with images and memories that are somehow tied into a habit cycle can trigger that cycle. Among the media triggers are:

Books
Television Commercials
Television Programs
Movies
Magazine Covers

PROBLEM AREA FIVE:
EMOTIONAL TRIGGERS

This is the largest category of triggers cited by addicted individuals. The power of emotional triggers is compounded by the fact that most of the particular emotions listed as triggers below can, in themselves, be addictive. Many of these triggers are also associated with triggers in other categories:

Boredom (This is the most common of all triggers.)
Depression
Anxieties and Stress
Feeling Overcommitted
Mental Exhaustion
Humiliation
Fear of Failure
Failure to Meet Obligations
The Agony of Defeat
Low Self-Esteem
Bitterness
Rejection
Envy
Jealousy

Resentment
Anger and Arguments
Desire to Make Up for Lost Time
Risk Taking
Feeling Challenged
Excitement
Fear of Success
Success
The Thrill of Victory
Happiness
Desire to Reward Oneself
Need to Consume and to Hoard
Feeling the Need to Experiment
Gambling With Oneself
Desire for New Identity
Search for Inner Peace
Confusion
Not Knowing What To Do
Feeling No Feelings *(No feeling is a feeling.)*

PROBLEM AREA SIX:
SPIRITUAL TRIGGERS

Many individuals suffering from detrimental addictive behaviors report a sense of spiritual malaise. Spiritual triggers, while addressing abstract and elusive feelings, are important in mapping addiction. Among these are:

Having No Values
Feeling A Void
Feeling of No Meaning in Life
Searching for Meaning
No Inner Peace
No Sense of Center
A Desire for Ritual
Replacing the Structured Religious Activity of Childhood With
an Adult Addiction

PROBLEM AREA SEVEN:
SOCIAL TRIGGERS

Interactions among pattern (drug, food, sex, spending, emotion, etc.) addicts and other individuals can stimulate addictive responses. Social triggers are numerous and interact with emotional, environmental, chemical, practical, and other triggers to strongly affect the addicted person. These include:

Peer Pressure
Drinking Buddies
Barhopping
Parties
Spectator Sporting Events
Business Lunches: you know the two martini lunch?
Workplace Interactions: fellow employees may share their alcohol and drugs with each other, or there maybe peer pressure to use drugs among co-workers. Co-workers may push other habits such as spending, eating, and sex pattern addictions.
Discussing One's Habit With Fellow Addicts: whether it be "war stories" or other forms of discussion, just talking about the addictive behavior can trigger it.
Association With Addicts: many addicts report that association with fellow addicts, fellow overeaters, or fellow druggers may trigger addictive behavior.
Association With Dealers: drug addicts may have within their social circles their "dealers" or "suppliers"—people from whom they buy or get their drugs. Overeaters may find their local restaurant, bakery, or deli owners playing the role of dealers.

Implicit addictions also respond to social triggers. Any social contact or experience which has been built into a holding or other energy pattern will serve as a kick-off point or trigger for that pattern.

PROBLEM AREA EIGHT:
PHYSICAL TRIGGERS

Temporary and permanent physical conditions are frequently unavoidable and often trigger addictive behavior. For example, among physical triggers are:

Trouble Waking Up in The Morning
Fatigue: tiredness, drowsiness, physical exhaustion.

Physical Depletion: that run-down feeling.

Lack of Exercise: this can lead to fatigue, trouble waking up, physical depletion, and a general malaise.

Pain: headaches, body aches, injuries.

Hunger: this can trigger all sorts of mood swngs.

Overeating: feeling full and fat.

Sexual Activity: anticipation, arousal, activity, postactivity.

Sensory Stimuli: such as the smell of the object of one's addiction, other odors, sounds, and sights. SENSORY TRIGGERS can easily become a separate category.

PROBLEM AREA NINE:
NUTRITIONAL TRIGGERS

Eating habits are a source of both obvious and hidden triggers. Eating fuels the body, and eating patterns fuel the body's energy patterns. The power of these nutritional triggers is compounded by the fact that eating itself can be addictive. These nutritional triggers include:

Irregular Eating
Overeating
Undereating
Not Eating
Empty Calorie, Junk Food Eating
Binge Eating
Nutritionally Imbalanced Eating

PROBLEM AREA TEN:
CHEMICAL TRIGGERS

Chemicals taken into the body may trigger a psychobiological chain of events leading an addicted individual to turn to the object of his addiction. When the addiction is to an emotional, behavioral, or energy pattern, mind- and body-altering chemicals such as those listed below can tie right into a cyclical habit pattern. When the object of addiction is a natural or artificial chemical (marijuana, alcohol, codeine, etc.), taken into the body in some way (via injection, eating, sniffing or smoking), the primary or explicit drug addiction is often triggered. Chemical triggers include:

Sugar
Nicotine
Caffeine
Alcohol
Marijuana
Cocaine
Other Illegal Drugs
Legal Drugs (Prescription and Nonprescription)
Poor Nutritional Food Combinations
Toxic Chemicals in the Workplace or Home
Environmental Irritants

Your list of triggers is actually never ending. In making a list such as the one above, you are brainstorming—searching your mind for as much information about yourself as you can possibly uncover. Be certain to write your list down on paper. Create more problem areas if that helps you to list more triggers. Vigilantly search yourself and your environment for both explicit (obvious) and implicit (hidden) triggers. The more triggers you write down, the more previously unrecognized triggers will float to the surface of your mind.

9

Trigger Charting: Seeing the Addiction Process

The pattern-addicted individuals who have identified their *general* problems (usually explicit addictions or health conditions), often feel overwhelmed by the task of identifying *specific* addictive patterns. The variables seem to be too numerous to identify. The addicted persons' behavioral idiosyncrasies may be entirely invisible to them at first, obscured by the perceived immensity of the problem. Once at least some of an addicted individual's triggers have been identified, the basic habit cycle or cycles can be dissected, diagrammed, and mapped, in order to better understand how they work.

To break a pattern addiction of any form, you must be able to clearly see how that addiction works. You must be able to call this awareness of the process into consciousness at any time. Mapping is one way to "see" this process. Mapping increases the level of awareness that you have of your process.

Mapping can be simple or complex, depending on the level of detail. All addictive behavior is multivariate; that is, a number of interrelated factors determine the behavior of the addicted individual. Usually the causes of an addictive behavior are so numerous and so inextricably linked that the roots of a particular addiction are difficult to pinpoint. The trigger chart described in this chapter is a powerful tool that helps "map out" addictive behavior. It is a personal behavioral inventory. The trigger chart allows you draw a profile of your trigger/response network.

Addiction is a confusing and uncertain territory. That is why, in the beginning, the trigger chart must be simple and clear. Triggers are elusive. When you first begin to identify yours, you may only spot one or two: "a fight with my spouse," or "social pressure to drink," for example. With proper guidance however, you will be able to map a much larger network of triggers.

The trigger chart is created by first defining problem areas in your life and then listing triggers (i.e., objects or events that bring out addictive behaviors) by their relevant category.

Mapping addictive behavior in this way enables you to "see" or define your condition. Gradually you will recognize, and add more triggers to, your chart. A trigger can be any experience, event, predicament, or impulse that sets off a chain of events leading to the manifesting of an addictive behavior. Anything can be a trigger, and every addicted individual has a unique set of triggers. These must be identified if you are to be able to work with the habitual response patterns that you have developed.

Once the process of trigger identification is started, many addicts report that it is never ending. Connected to every trigger are other triggers. Behind and connected to every obvious, explicit trigger is a web of less obvious, implicit triggers. For example, a refrigerator full of delicious desserts may trigger an overeater into an eating binge. Behind this explicit trigger, the refrigerator, is a network of other triggers which are either entirely unacknowledged or are lingering on the edge of the overeating addict's awareness. An argument with a spouse may trigger a bout of chronic back pain. The argument is the explicit trigger, but a web of tensions, energy blocks, physical injuries, and emotional memories compose a set of interlinked, networked, implicit triggers.

Whatever your addictions may be, the process of mapping your pattern addictions becomes an investigation into your entire lifestyle. Once the unwieldy problem of addictive dependence is diagrammed and dissected, it *can* be understood. It can slowly be unearthed and brought to your awareness. One must *see* the cycle of detrimental patterning in order to break it. As was pointed out before, a *trigger* stimulates your *urge* to manifest your addictive behavior. When you give in to your urge you are experiencing the addictive *response* to that urge. Prior to the detailed identification of your triggers, you experience such urges without insight into the intricate web of causality leading to them. But once you understand the pattern or cycle, you can break that cycle at any of its three points: at the trigger point, the urge point, or the response point. Understanding your addiction cycle begins with identifying your triggers. This is how you create a trigger chart:

MAPPING AN ADDICTION

Step One: Begin to List Your Triggers

This is a brainstorming process. Uncovering memories and ideas will take the lock off the door to your mind. For every trigger identified, there will be at least one, if not several, other triggers that come to mind. Over time, other triggers will surface into your consciousness, as if lifting the obvious triggers by listing them allows implicit triggers to float to the surface of your consciousness. List everything that comes to mind in all or most of the following categories:

PRACTICAL TRIGGERS
TEMPORAL TRIGGERS
ENVIRONMENTAL TRIGGERS
MEDIA TRIGGERS
EMOTIONAL TRIGGERS
SPIRITUAL TRIGGERS
SOCIAL TRIGGERS
PHYSICAL TRIGGERS
NUTRITIONAL TRIGGERS
CHEMICAL TRIGGERS
OTHER CATEGORIES OF TRIGGERS

Refer to Chapter 8 for examples of triggers within many of these categories. Recognize that these categories overlap. They are listed separately to stimulate your brainstorming. Work with a large piece of paper, perhaps an 18″ by 24″ sheet of butcher paper. Try to use a different colored felt-tip pen for each category. List as many triggers as you can think of in each of these categories. Some triggers will fit into more than one or into no category. Write these triggers down anywhere you like.

Step Two: Add Triggers to Your List

Add at least five triggers in each category. If this is difficult, think in terms of primary (explicit and obvious), secondary (less explicit and less obvious), and tertiary (very implicit and very hidden) triggers. For example, cocaine addicts will find that a pile of cocaine is a primary trigger. A secondary trigger for them might be an empty plastic bag of the sort that they have used to store their cocaine. A tertiary or incidental trigger might be something that reminds them of either the primary trigger, say a pile of sugar, or of the secondary trigger, perhaps a clear piece of plastic. Another and more implicit tertiary trigger might be a drop in energy caused by a shift in blood sugar level, or a mood swing related to some family problem. That drop in energy and mood swing into depression may stimulate a craving for the cocaine, which is a stimulant.

However you go about your brainstorming, be sure to write down *anything* that comes to mind, no matter how trivial. Any association at all is ripe material for the trigger chart. Do not try to make sense out of everything. Just let it all come into your awareness and write it all down. Write as quickly as you can without trying to be neat. You can clean up your list and organize it later.

Once you have listed everything that you can think of, draw a box or a circle around each individual trigger.

Step Three: Connect Your Triggers to Form Patterns

Now examine all of your triggers. Do you feel that any of them are connected? Draw a line between these triggers. Some connections will seem logical, others will seem to make no sense at all. For example, at five o'clock Friday (a time trigger) Bill, a person addicted to the drug alcohol, may go to a particular bar (an environmental trigger) where he may see Mark and Sally (social triggers), feel like partying (a psychological trigger), and eat a large amount of salty nuts and potato chips instead of a real dinner because he is hungry but too lazy to eat right (a nutritional trigger). And after all that salt he may be so thirsty that he finally "breaks down" (probably a state of mind, a psychological trigger driven by a physical or psychological trigger) and has a beer (a chemical trigger), which leads to several more drinks (more chemical triggers), each of which invites the next drink.

This is a fairly obvious pattern. Other patterns will be less clear, but any patterns that come to mind should be recorded. People who are addicted to drugs (including alcohol, nicotine, and caffeine) often experience triggers that seem inexplicable at first glance. For example, the smell of flowers may remind you of the incense you once used to cover the smell of marijuana, which, in turn, reminds you of other drugs. However, you may, at first, just see that the smell of the flowers leads to a craving for drugs. Or a favorite song may make you want to have a glass of wine. Or the smell of a cigarette burning may lead you to want to smell marijuana smoke. Or the sound that a knife makes on a cutting board as you chop vegetables may remind you of chopping a line of cocaine with a razor blade.

If you are working on a chart of a more subtle, implicit pattern, you will have to be even more open to the seemingly random associations your mind makes. For example, if you have a habit of pulling out your hair strand by strand or lash by lash, you may assume that you do this automatically and have no triggers. However, upon study, you may find that having nothing, or nothing of interest, to do with your hands is a trigger. You may also discover that you only do this when you are alone. If you have digestive problems such as an ulcer or a preulcerous condition, you may think that this problem arises when you eat spicy food and when you are under stress. Yet you can dissect these too explicit triggers into the many triggers that they really are: many foods and multiple stressors. You may also eventually discover that you rarely breathe deeply and that you hold your abdominal area tense without realizing that you are doing so. Holding this area tense results in pressure on, and reduced blood flow to, the digestive organs.

Whatever your pattern addictions may be, continue to map out relationships among the various triggers you have listed. Observe the patterns that emerge. The charts at the end of this chapter are actually simple maps of several different addicted individuals' "habit territories." Notice the similarities and differences in these charts.

Your addiction chart should be reconstructed regularly. Add to your first chart daily for a week. Make a new chart each week for ten weeks, incorporating everything from your old chart and pushing yourself to add new details. For the next ten months, make a new chart once a month. Then shift to two or three times a year. This will provide you with an amazing journey into your behavior and a new level of awareness about yourself.

In the beginning, you may focus on one habit at a time, such as a drug habit or an overeating habit. Later, when you feel comfortable with the basic trigger mapping, you may want to draw two or more charts on a giant piece of paper and look for connections among your addictions. You may want to begin with the most obvious, explicit addictions that you feel you have and then move to your more implicit addictions as you find them.

Whenever you find connections among triggers, draw lines to demonstrate those connections. Long after some of your more explicit patterns have diminished (and they will if you so desire), this mapping process will reveal significant information about your emotional, behavioral, and energetic patterns.

I have included sample trigger charts here. The first four (Figures 9.1–9.4) were done by people explicitly addicted to drugs who were just learning to chart. Figures 9.5 and 9.6 are somewhat more implicit. Figure

9.5 is an early search for implicit triggers behind a young man's chronic nausea and headaches. Figure 9.6 is a middle-aged woman's effort to delve into an ongoing feeling of general malaise and illness that she fears is going to lead to serious illness. Figure 9.7 is a more detailed chart done, with my help, by a multiple drug user who had been studying charting for some time. Although these charts are presented in a top-to-bottom fashion, many people I have worked with have chosen to draw their charts in a circular form. As you repeat the charting process for your own pattern addictions, your own chart will gain details and levels. Its format (linear or circular) may change. Eventually, you will draw something more complex than any of these charts. Examine Figures 9.5 and 9.6 for hints of more implicit addiction patterns. In Chapters 11 and 12 we will examine other routes to the discovery of intricate habit patterning deep within the psyche.

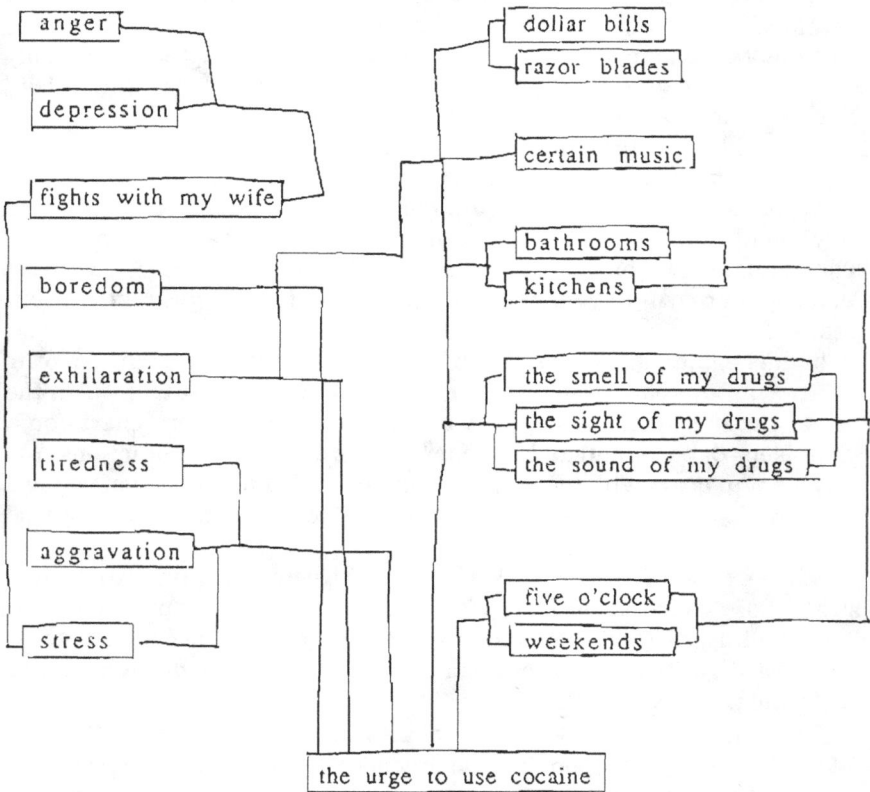

Figure 9.1. Sample Trigger Chart #1

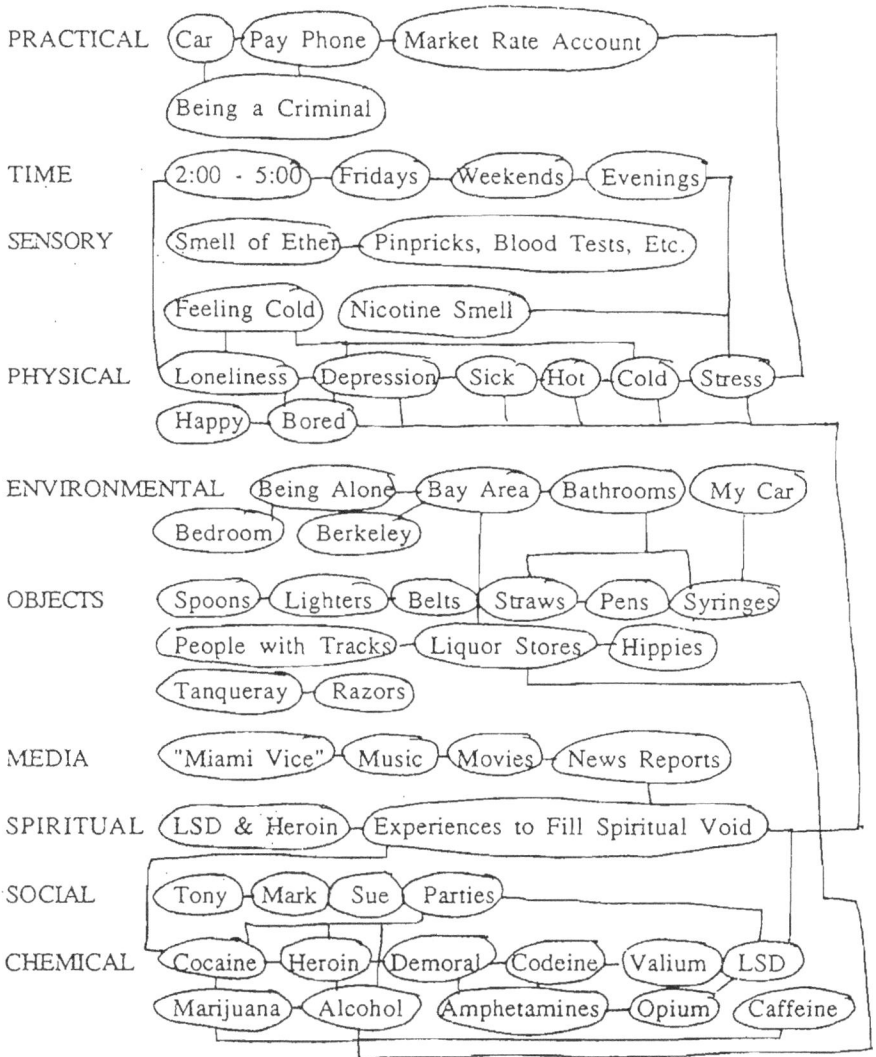

Figure 9.2. Sample Trigger Chart #2

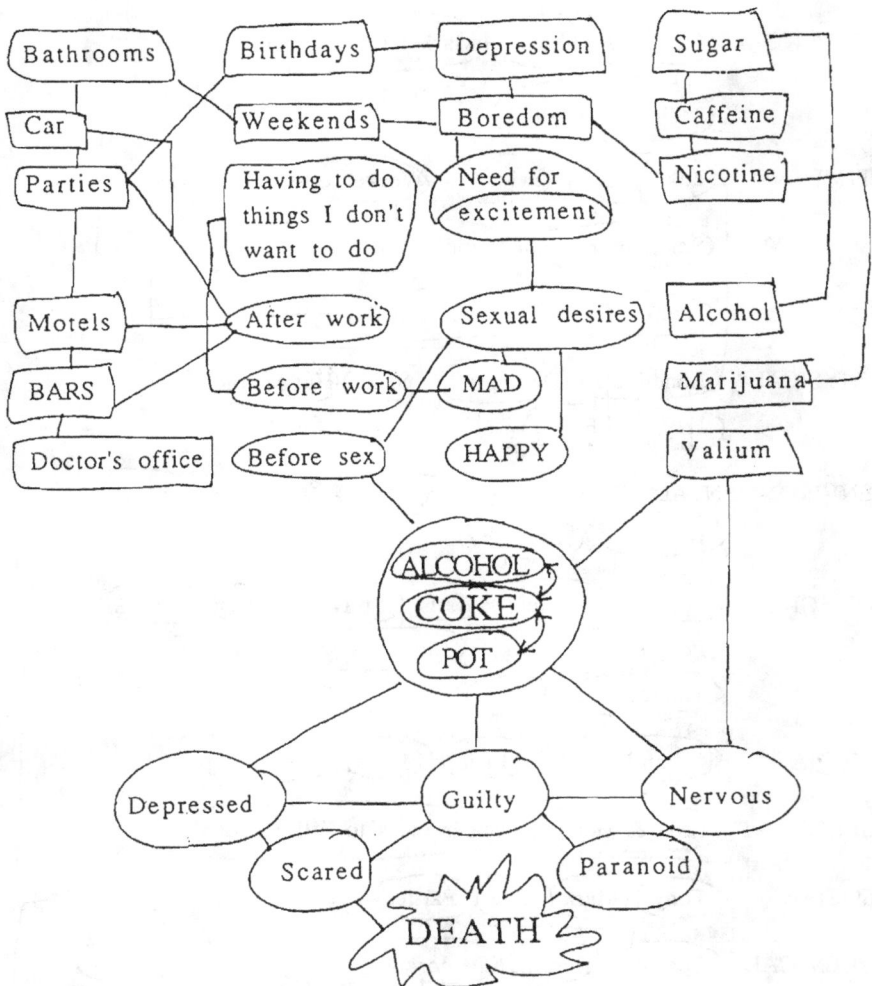

Figure 9.3. Sample Trigger Chart #3

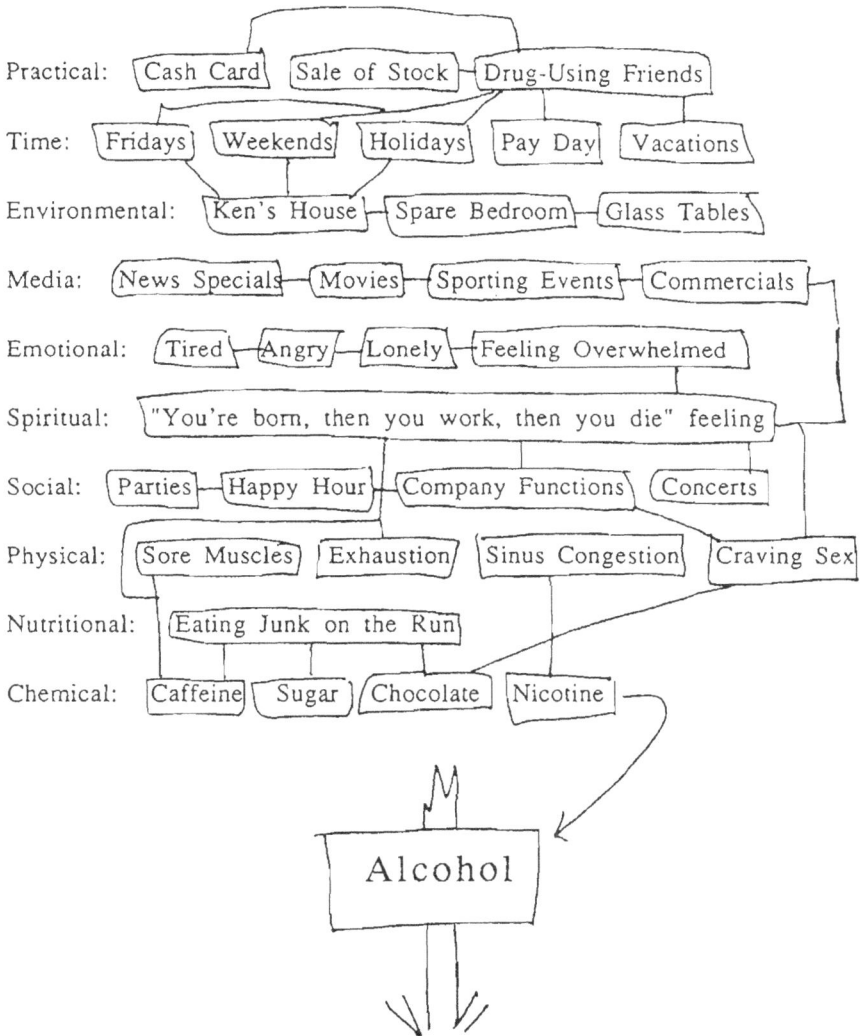

Practical: Cash Card | Sale of Stock | Drug-Using Friends

Time: Fridays | Weekends | Holidays | Pay Day | Vacations

Environmental: Ken's House | Spare Bedroom | Glass Tables

Media: News Specials | Movies | Sporting Events | Commercials

Emotional: Tired | Angry | Lonely | Feeling Overwhelmed

Spiritual: "You're born, then you work, then you die" feeling

Social: Parties | Happy Hour | Company Functions | Concerts

Physical: Sore Muscles | Exhaustion | Sinus Congestion | Craving Sex

Nutritional: Eating Junk on the Run

Chemical: Caffeine | Sugar | Chocolate | Nicotine

Alcohol

Figure 9.4. Sample Trigger Chart #4

Practical: Convenience of Old Ways of Being

Time: No Time to Concentrate on Self

Nutritional: Carbohydrate Overuse   Eating Irregularly   Fatty Foods

Physical: No Sleep   Exhaustion   Poor Digestion   Ulcers   Overweight

Energetic: Tightness in Neck, Jaw and Stomach

Emotional: Hopelessness   Sense of No Control Over Life

Spiritual: Emptiness   Meaninglessness

SICK FEELING

and

HEADACHES ALL THE TIME

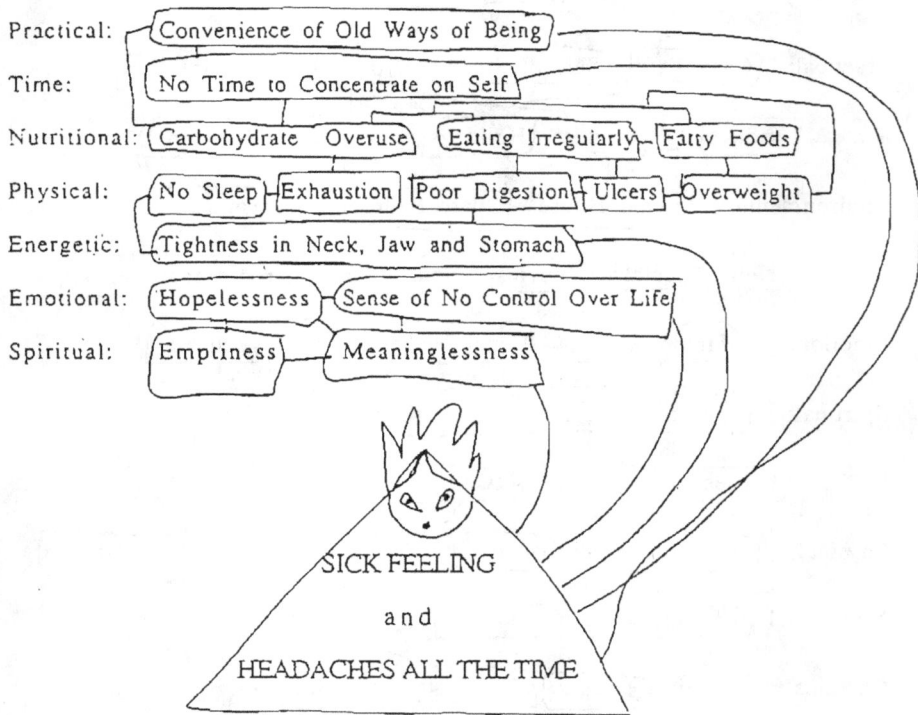

Figure 9.5.   Sample Trigger Chart #5

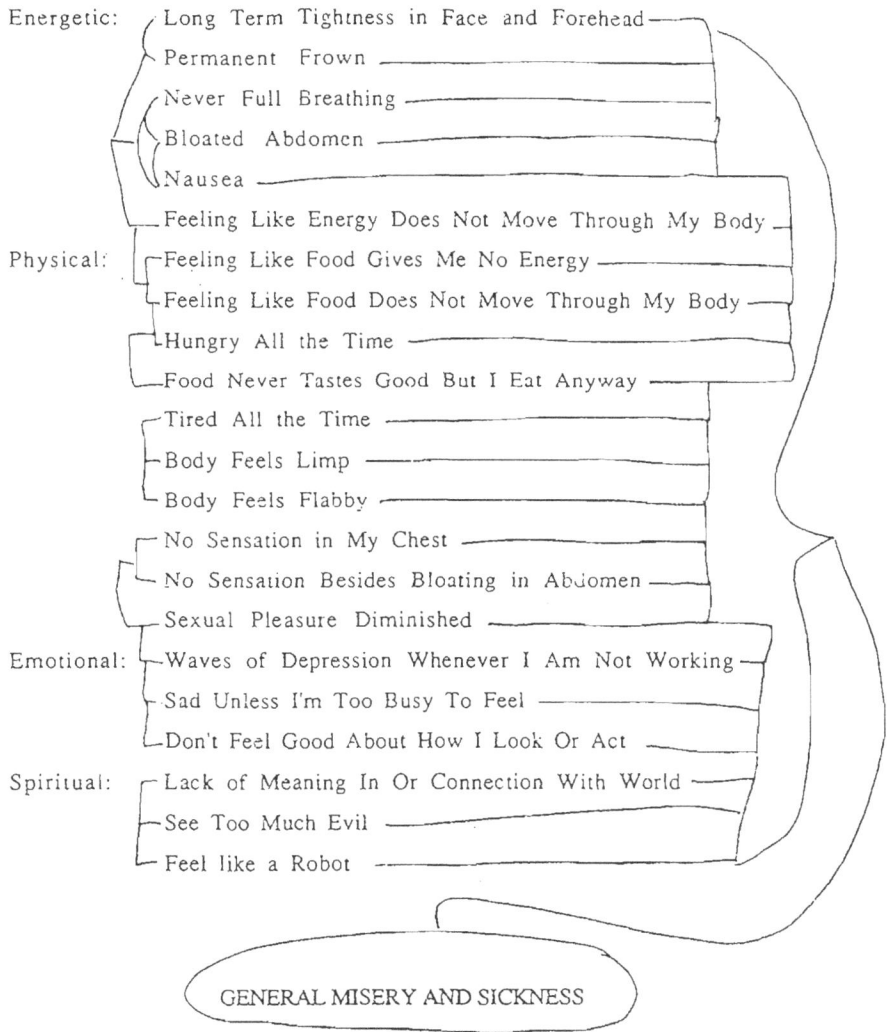

Energetic:
- Long Term Tightness in Face and Forehead
- Permanent Frown
- Never Full Breathing
- Bloated Abdomen
- Nausea

Physical:
- Feeling Like Energy Does Not Move Through My Body
- Feeling Like Food Gives Me No Energy
- Feeling Like Food Does Not Move Through My Body
- Hungry All the Time
- Food Never Tastes Good But I Eat Anyway
- Tired All the Time
- Body Feels Limp
- Body Feels Flabby
- No Sensation in My Chest
- No Sensation Besides Bloating in Abdomen
- Sexual Pleasure Diminished

Emotional:
- Waves of Depression Whenever I Am Not Working
- Sad Unless I'm Too Busy To Feel
- Don't Feel Good About How I Look Or Act

Spiritual:
- Lack of Meaning In Or Connection With World
- See Too Much Evil
- Feel like a Robot

GENERAL MISERY AND SICKNESS

Figure 9.6. Sample Trigger Chart #6

ADDICTION TRIGGER CHART ©

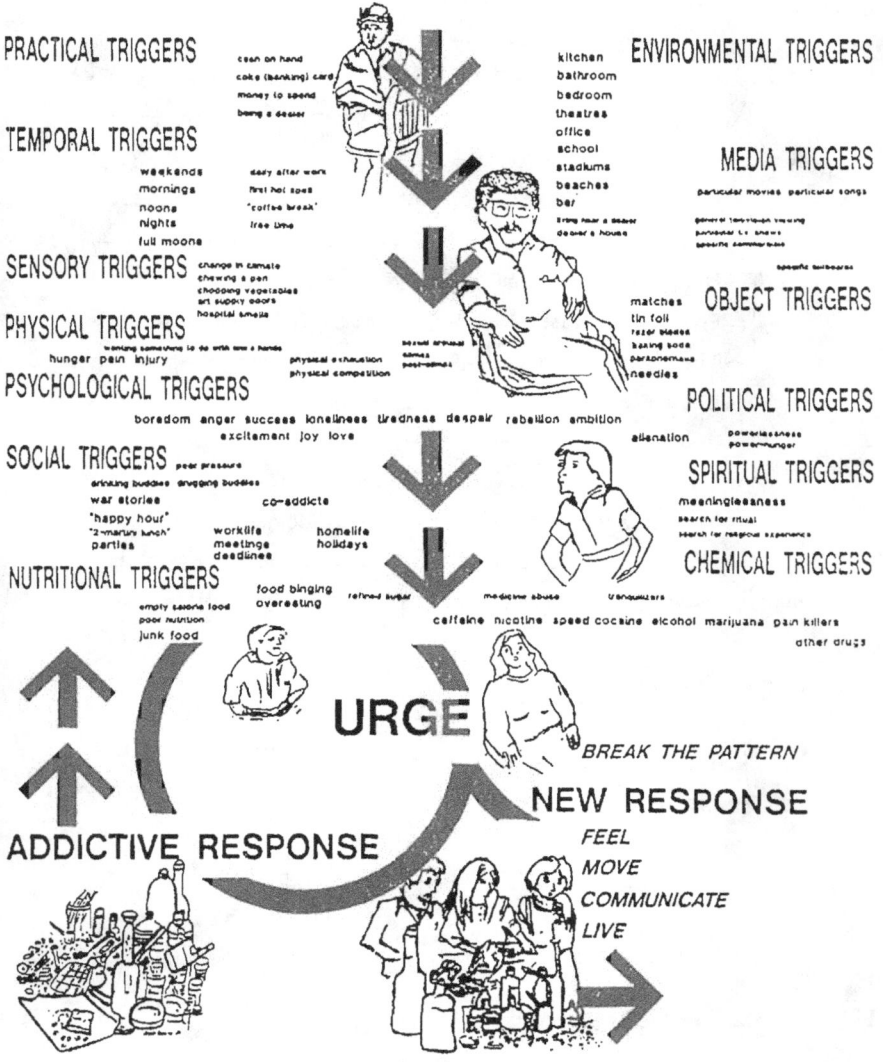

PRACTICAL TRIGGERS
cash on hand
cards (banking) card
money to spend
being a dealer

ENVIRONMENTAL TRIGGERS
kitchen
bathroom
bedroom
theatres
office
school
stadiums
beaches
bar

TEMPORAL TRIGGERS
weekends
mornings
noons
nights
full moons

daily after work
first hot spell
"coffee break"
free time

being near a dealer
dealer's house

MEDIA TRIGGERS
particular movies particular songs

general television viewing
particular t.v. shows
specific commercials

specific billboards

SENSORY TRIGGERS
change in climate
chewing a pen
chopping vegetables
art supply odors
hospital smells

OBJECT TRIGGERS
matches
tin foil
razor blades
baking soda
paraphernalia
needles

PHYSICAL TRIGGERS
hunger pain injury
wanting something to do with one's hands
physical exhaustion
physical competition

sexual arousal
games
post-orgasm

PSYCHOLOGICAL TRIGGERS
boredom anger success loneliness tiredness despair rebellion ambition
excitement joy love

POLITICAL TRIGGERS
alienation
powerlessness
power-hunger

SOCIAL TRIGGERS peer pressure
drinking buddies drugging buddies
war stories
"happy hour"
"2-martini lunch"
parties

co-addicte

worklife
meetings
deadlines

homelife
holidays

SPIRITUAL TRIGGERS
meaninglessness
search for ritual
search for religious experience

NUTRITIONAL TRIGGERS
empty calorie food
poor nutrition
junk food

food binging
overeating

refined sugar

CHEMICAL TRIGGERS

medicine abuse tranquilizers

caffeine nicotine speed cocaine alcohol marijuana pain killers
other drugs

URGE

BREAK THE PATTERN

NEW RESPONSE
FEEL
MOVE
COMMUNICATE
LIVE

ADDICTIVE RESPONSE

Figure 9.7.   Sample Trigger Chart #7

80

10

Life Management Planning: How to Live Well

Once your triggers have been clearly identified, they can be changed or avoided. This takes a lot of work and a lot of commitment. Mostly it takes solid *life management planning*.

Fix the following principle in your mind:

TRANSCENDING
PATTERN ADDICTION
is a
WILLINGNESS TO DO SOMETHING NEW
to make a
COMMITMENT
to
HARD WORK
on many levels, including the:
PRACTICAL
PHYSICAL
NUTRITIONAL
CHEMICAL
ENVIRONMENTAL
SOCIAL
PSYCHOLOGICAL
ENERGETIC
and
SPIRITUAL
LEVELS OF BEING.

This is what I call *lifestyle surgery*. Hard work on only one level results in change on only one level; and, change on one level is not enough to overpower the force of any pattern addiction. Holistic change is necessary. This takes a combination of close scrutiny of every level of your life and a marked effort to change on all of these levels. The following multilevel *Life Management Plan* is a practical fleshing-out of the program for lifestyle surgery described in Chapter 7. It is a sound, methodological program for change. You may want to begin the plan, one segment at a time, adding a new level to your life management each week. Write yourself a schedule sheet to keep track of your progress. Schedule in advance the dates on which you will add a new level to your plan. A careful following of this plan will enable you to change or avoid your triggers and break the cycle of detrimental pattern addiction. Whether you are working on an explicit or an implicit addiction, the matter of life management is critical. Learning to organize and to be highly conscious of one's exterior reality is essential training for spiritual progress. (Spiritual progress occurs in one's interior reality.)

A LIFE MANAGEMENT PLAN

Set up one or more three-ring binders with as many dividers as you need to organize the ongoing notes you will make in each of the following categories.

THE PRACTICAL LEVEL

Time Management

Time and *time* again, poor *time* management leads people back into the storm of addiction. Commit yourself to developing time management skills by continuously tracking, and then improving through careful planning, the use of your time.

> ORGANIZE YOUR LIFE MANAGEMENT PLAN by writing a long term schedule or calendar which designates days and times for beginning and continuing each segment of this plan.
>
> KEEP A SLEEP DIARY of every time you sleep, whether it be a nap or your night's rest, during each week. Evaluate and amend these times to implement the following goals:

- *Regularity:* Go to sleep and wake up at approximately the same time every day. Also, if you nap, try to nap at the same time every day.
- *Adequacy:* Get enough sleep. Enough is variable. If you already know what constitutes a good level of sleep for you, aim for that level. While not everyone sleeps eight hours a night, this is a healthy average to aim for if you are uncertain about your own needs.
- *Satisfaction:* If you feel sleepy, you either need more sleep, more exercise, better nutrition, or perhaps have some other physical of psychological need. Aim for a deep sense of satisfaction with your sleep habits. Other elements of this life management plan may also help to reduce your fatigue.

KEEP A DAILY RECORD OF YOUR SCHEDULE FOR A MONTH. Record everything that you do and note how long you do each activity. Once you have an accurate picture of your schedule, evaluate and amend it to incorporate the following goals:

- *Regularity:* Live a life with a regular and predictable pace to it.
- *Variety within the free time periods:* Although you want to achieve a regular and predictable pace to your life, build in regular free time periods that include a variety of recreational activities.
- *Adequacy in terms of health-promotion:* Examine your schedule for its intensity. Find a reasonable midpoint between days with a sluggish pace and days that are *over*booked.
- *Utility in your addiction-affliction recovery process:* Be certain your schedule leaves room for and includes specific therapy sessions and other prescribed activities that are essential to overcoming your addictions and other health problems.
- *Satisfaction:* Develop a sense of satisfaction with each day of your life. Continue for one or more years to consciously revise your daily schedule to achieve this. One way to track your level of satisfaction is to review each day for five minutes each night before falling asleep. This review also helps you become more conscious of the time of your life and how you are spending it on a day-to-day basis.

KEEP A RECORD OF HOW YOU SPEND YOUR FREE TIME. Write down how long you do which free-time activities each day, the initials of the person with whom you did those things, and any items of particular interest for that day. Then evaluate and amend these times for:

- *Effects upon your recovery:* Be careful not to use your free time in ways that will trigger further urges to manifest your explicit addictions such as overeating or drug or alcohol using. Examine your free time for friends, places and experiences that may trigger your addictive behavior. *(Remember, these people do not actually trigger your behaviors, but you may react to them as if they do.)*
- *Pleasure derived:* Are you enjoying your free time? Your free time is valuable and should be used effectively. Look around. Find pleasurable and healthy free-time activities.
- *Satisfaction:* Aim to feel satisfaction with the use of your free time.
- *Learning:* Learn as much as you can about what *free time* means to you. We are all different. No one else can tell you what will feel free to you.

REMEMBER TO ALWAYS:

- *Plan ahead:* Do not leave yourself open to automatic addictive behavior by leaving unplanned hours and days.
- *Have back up plans:* Be certain that you have other options in case a date is cancelled or plans fall through. Not having a back-up plan can trigger addictive behavior.
- *Do not change your schedule on the spur of the moment:* This means just what is says: Do *not* change your schedule on the spur of the moment. You can easily succumb to addictive patterns this way.
- *Build useful activities into your lifestyle on all levels:* Be sure to plan to sleep, eat, exercise, work, take time for yourself, call or see friends who know that you are working to transcend your addiction, and do whatever else your doctor, therapist, counselor, or other advisor (if you have one) has prescribed for you. Write these and other activities into your weekly schedule.

Money Management

The ability to organize one's money—using spending, budgeting, and savings skills, can bring about confidence in the material world. This is not about the size of one's income; this is about the sense of self-awareness that comes through monitoring one's economic participation.

KEEP A MONEY DIARY of daily spending and saving for one week. Leave *no* loan or purchase out of the diary. Then evaluate your spending and savings habits by the following criteria.

- *Sense of Control:* If you find that you have trouble handling "cash on hand" (in your hands, pockets, wallet, drawers, etc.), arrange ways to not have cash or get hold of it easily. Gain a sense of control over your use of money by doing what it takes to make it difficult to spend money on your habit or in response to emotional or other triggers. Pinpoint all the areas in which you have money management difficulties: paydays, credit cards, automated teller machine cards, cash on hand, compulsive spending. Be certain to come up with a plan for, or seek counseling regarding, each difficulty. Bookkeepers, accountants, and financial counselors can be helpful.
- *Useful spending:* Decide what expenditures are essential (such as rent, food, and taxes). Then decide what expenditures are necessary in your fight to transcend your addictive behavior. Note your many unessential expenditures. Prioritize your spending categories.

BUDGET. Write a budget for each month before the month begins. Stick to your budget for that month. Do not make changes during the month. If you think that you've budgeted too little or too much for a particular item, do not change midmonth. Unless you have a life-threatening emergency, wait and amend next month's budget. Notice when, and under what emotional conditions, you have trouble sticking to your budget. This is especially important for spending, credit card use, shopping, and gambling addicts.

THE PHYSICAL LEVEL

Exercise Management

If you do not manage your body, it will manage you. Take control. A healthy body has fewer cravings for the consumption of unnecessary and unhealthy food and drugs and for doing other self-destructive activities. And, awareness of physical health reflects itself in awareness of psychological well-being.

SEE YOUR DOCTOR for advice regarding the appropriate exercises for your age and physical condition. Do this immediately.

KEEP A LIST OF ALL EXERCISE that you perform each week: the types of exercise, the times of day, and their durations.

EVALUATE AND AMEND THIS LIST for:

- *Regularity:* Regular exercise, as approved by your doctor if you are or should be under medical supervision, is a must.
- *Adequacy:* Be certain to select exercises that suit your level of physical health. Be certain to get enough exercise, without overexercising. If you have never exercised before, begin with a leisurely twenty-minute walk each day. Even a very brisk thirty- to sixty-minute walk four times a week can be excellent exercise. If you have a heart condition, or if you experience shortness of breath or dizziness when you walk or jog, see a physician. Whatever your level of athletic ability, avoid sports injuries; these can lead to or trigger a recycling back into full expression of your pattern addiction.
- *Satisfaction:* Strive for satisfaction with your physical exercises. Try different exercises until you find those that fit your temperament and tastes.

Hygiene Management

Stay clean. This may seem an extraneous activity, but the upkeep of your personal hygiene is a vital key to the upkeep your self-respect and self-image.

TAKE A LOOK AT YOURSELF and note any areas of your body that you feel could use some attention, i.e., your fingernails, your gums, your hair, your skin. Learn to improve and take care of these trouble spots.

BUILD HYGIENE INTO YOUR SCHEDULE. Write personal hygiene into your weekly plan, even if you feel that you are already a hygienic person.

THE NUTRITIONAL LEVEL

Nutritional Management

Caring about yourself means caring about what you put into yourself. Manage what you eat and you will learn to manage a lot of other areas of your life. Nutritional imbalances can affect your energy, your emotions, your addictive behaviors, your health, and your attention span.

EAT REGULARLY.

EAT BALANCED.

EAT ENOUGH.

EAT NOTHING IN EXCESS.

EAT CALORIES WITH NUTRITIONAL VALUE.

KNOW WHAT YOU EAT. Ask yourself and write down the answers to these questions:

- *What did I eat and drink yesterday?*
- *What did I eat and drink each day of last week?*

  for breakfast, if anything?
  for a morning snack?
  for lunch?
  during the afternoon?
  for dinner?
  for desert?
  for a midnight snack?

ARRANGE THE ANSWERS TO THESE QUESTIONS INTO THE CATEGORIES LISTED ON THE FOOD CONSUMPTION CHART. Now, in order to do something with your answers to the above questions, Xerox (or copy by hand) the food consumption chart on the next page. (If you do Xerox it, make several copies while you are at it—start with thirty to fifty of them.) Try to rearrange the answers you wrote to the above questions for all, or even just one, of the days you wrote about onto a copy of the food consumption chart. Put the different food items you consumed into the categories listed below. You may list a food more than once if you feel that its ingredients fit more than one category.

KEEP A RECORD OF WHAT YOU EAT by listing *every*thing you eat and the time of day you eat it on the food consumption chart. The best way to see your eating behavior is to this for at least one full month. Some people choose to do it for at least a year, or for one month every few months for many years, in order to maintain a high level of awareness about what they put into their bodies. When you do keep the list, leave no day and no food off of the list. Include all snacks and any empty calorie foods as well as all nutritious items. Use the back of the page or extra list pages if you need more room to be thorough. Also note your mood, location, and other information about what is going on when you eat that food.

Food Consumption Chart

Date: _____

Time: _____

| FOOD GROUPS | MOOD | LOCATION | NOTES |

MEAT, POULTRY and FISH

- -
- -
- -

DAIRY PRODUCTS

- -
- -

FRUITS and VEGETABLES

- -
- -

NUTS and GRAINS

- -
- -

EMPTY CALORIE, "JUNK" FOODS

- -
- -

SALT

- -
- -

SUGAR

- -
- -

CAFFEINE

- -
- -

ALCOHOL

- -
- -

OTHER DRUGS

- -
- -

OTHER FOOD ADDITIVES

- -
- -
- -

IMPROVE YOUR EATING by evaluating your eating habits for:

- *Regularity:* Try to eat and snack at approximately the same times each day.
- *Balance:* Begin by eliminating your overeating in one or two of the food groups. First cut down on salt, for example, then on empty calorie, nonnutritious junk foods. Survey your eating habits for undereating and irregular eating as well as for overeating. Be aware of your eating patterns and pinpoint changes that you want to make in them.
- *Food Groups:* Eat food from each of the following five food groups every day: nuts and grains, vegetables, fruits, dairy products, and fish/poultry/meat. If you are a vegetarian, leave out the fish, poultry, and meat food group, but be sure to achieve a balanced protein intake. Work with a nutritionist if you are uninformed in the area of dietary health.
- *Water:* Be certain you drink at least eight 8 ounce glasses of water each day. This is a lot of water, but it really helps your body to function more smoothly. Drinking water helps to control weight, water retention, and the pile-up of wastes.
- *Empty Calorie Eating:* Examine your food intake for the presence of drugs and additives, fast foods, junk foods and foods that have a high salt or sugar content. Stop eating foods whose calories carry little nutritional value.
- *Satisfaction:* Seek to feel satisfied and happy with what you eat. Search for healthy meals that you can enjoy.

THE CHEMICAL LEVEL

Chemical and Craving Management

This book has used drug addiction as its primary example of explicit addiction. Drug and food addictions can also be implicit addictions when they are not recognized as explicit addictions. Far too many of us live with little and big drug and food addictions and fail to realize this. Whether or not you think you are addicted to drugs (including alcohol, caffeine, nicotine, prescription drugs, and over-the-counter drugs), or food:

NOTE ALL CRAVINGS that you experience for alcohol, caffeine, nicotine other drugs, or foods. Every time you experience a craving, even a mild craving, note down the:

- *day*
- *time*

- *duration*
- *object of craving*
- *how you respond to the craving*
- *how you could respond differently to this craving.*

PLAN NEW RESPONSES. When you discover a hitherto unrecognized craving, study it. Whether they be new or old cravings or urges, think of ways you could respond differently to them, such as calling a friend, taking a walk, beating a pillow, eating a healthy meal. Incorporate these new responses into your weekly schedule—build them into your life by writing them into the schedule in anticipation of future cravings. Plan these responses ahead of time to break the habit cycle and get out of automatic mode

THE ENVIRONMENTAL LEVEL

Living Environment Management

A clean, organized, and attractive living environment is a manageable living environment. Your physical world is, or can be, a representation of your emotional world.

EVALUATE YOUR ENVIRONMENT for its:

- *Cleanliness*
- *Organization*
- *Attractiveness*
- *Comfort*

IMPROVE YOUR ENVIRONMENT ON A REGULAR BASIS in each of the above categories. Expensive, radical changes are not always necessary. Simply make a continual effort to make small improvements.

Environmental Triggers Management

Many physical objects, large and small, serve to trigger the addicted individual's addictive behavior.

IDENTIFY THE PHYSICAL TRIGGERS IN YOUR ENVIRONMENT. Analyze the affects that particular objects and places have on you.

WHEN NECESSARY, REMOVE THESE TRIGGERS from your environment.

THE SOCIAL LEVEL

Family Life Management

Family life changes when one or more members of the family decide to break their addictions. Because all family members are affected by your decision to transcend addiction, you should include all your family members in your

> TIME MANAGEMENT,
> MONEY MANAGEMENT,
> NUTRITIONAL MANAGEMENT PLANNING,
> OTHER MANAGEMENT AREAS RELEVANT TO THE FAMILY.

Work Life Management

Work life is a central element of many addictive patterns. Evaluate and amend your work life to

> CONTROL WORK-RELATED TRIGGERS.
> SUSTAIN WORK LIFE WITHOUT BEING OVERCOME BY IT.
> FIND SATISFACTION IN YOUR WORK.

General Social Life Management

Certain friends and social activities are likely to pull an addicted individual back into the snare of his addictive behavior. Manage your social life to

> AVOID OR RISE ABOVE SOCIAL OR PEER PRESSURE (pressure to resume your addictive behavior),
> GENERATE POSITIVE SOCIAL CONTACT,
> FIND SOCIAL SUPPORT,
> ENJOY HEALTHY SOCIAL TIME.

THE PSYCHOLOGICAL LEVEL

Emotion Management

Feel and fully express the pain and confusion of addiction, and the joy and fulfillment of rising above addiction. Do not shut these emotions out. Do not ignore them. Do not feel that, if your addiction is implicit, you have nothing to express. Give full voice to any feelings you have in this process. Tell friends, write in a diary, talk to a tape recorder, have someone make a video tape of you, or talk to a psychotherapist or other counselor.

Commitment Management

Fully decide to transcend your addiction. Experience the many setbacks and successes that are a part of this process. You must always strive to *believe in yourself*. As discussed in Chapter 4 and in this chapter under "The Spiritual Level," develop the ability to:

DECIDE TO BE COMMITTED
FEEL COMMITTED
FEEL COMMITTED ON ALL LEVELS

Stress Management

Stress is the result of an unresolved problem or an incomplete development. The lack of resolution and completion creates tension. Sometimes this tension is healthy and growth promoting, but sometimes stress can make you nervous, ill at ease, sick, and perhaps even kill you.

> KNOW STRESS. There is no way· around stress. Every profound life change is stressful. This means that even a change for the better, such as stopping a destructive pattern addiction, generates stress. You may have adapted to the stress of your addiction so thoroughly that you may not even recognize it as stress. But when new stresses—typical of healthy change and the growing pains of transcendence—appear, you feel their impact because they are new. You may even feel afraid of this newly recognized stress. However, this stress can be used well by turning this tension into valuable, productive energy. *good stress management is essential.*

RECOGNIZE STRESS AS AN OPPORTUNITY. Stress is always taking place in our lives. Our response to that stress determines whether we will become ill or turn it into a chance to master the challenges of life. Addiction offers this opportunity to those who recognize it. To begin healing your addiction, manage your stress, or to a photograph of that person.

- *Remember that life can be stressful:* Addiction is stressful. And recovery from addiction is stressful.
- *Identify stressful events in your individual and family history:* Be certain to discuss them with a counselor or therapist. Comb your emotional make-up and the store-house of your heart to identify, and then express and work through, any unresolved feelings you find.
- *Stay current with your feelings:* Check yourself out at the end of each day. Ask yourself, "Are there any unexpressed feelings that I am carrying?" If there are, make a note about them, and then cry, yell, laugh—express them. If you are angry at someone, find a healthy way to express your anger to that person, or to a photograph of that person.
- *Identify stressors as they appear:* Pay close attention to your physical reactions to them. Are you grinding your teeth, perspiring, salivating, aching, twitching? Is your heart pounding? Are you breathing rapidly or gasping for air? Sometimes your body will recognize that you are feeling stress before your mind does. Sometimes your mind will not recognize your body recognizing stress until you teach it how to. Ask your mind to pay attention in detail to your body.
- *When you identify a stressor or a symptom of stress, take measures:*
  Focus on the physical symptoms, whether they be vague or profound,
  Concentrate on your breathing,
  Do some physical exercise or stretching, if you can,
  Call a friend.
- *Always remember that life is stressful at every turning point:* There is no way to avoid stress, but honest communication and a good social support system, combined with exercise, good nutrition, and paying attention to emotions, do a lot to reduce stress.

- *Remember the opportunities that stress provides:* Stress gives us all a chance to master the challenge of life. It is not a challenge we can macho, bulldoze through, or overpower. We must learn to feel and listen and share. When we master and then overcome negative responses to stress, we gain the strength, power, and understanding that will propel us forward on our journey of transcendence. Stress can be used as jet power fuel for personal growth.

THE ENERGETIC LEVEL

Pattern Recognition Management

Write a new trigger chart (see Chapter 9) for yourself each week, trying not to consult your old one and trying to dig deeper, adding more explicit and implicit triggers each time.

Pattern Repair Management

Do the exercises provided in Chapters 11 and 12 at least twice a week for the first month and then continue on a weekly basis. After a few months, continue only with the exercise in Chapter 12. Note how you improve at this esoteric exercise over time.

THE SPIRITUAL LEVEL

Condition Management

Practice the exercises provided in Chapter Four. Use the schedule provided in that chapter for a least half a year.

    COMMITMENT
    ATTENTION
    FORTITUDE
    FAITH

Phase Management

Learn to recognize which phases of transcendence you have been through and which phases you are presently in, as explained in Chapter 4. Remember, these are:

PHASE 1: STRUGGLE
PHASE 2: PARADOX
PHASE 3: INSIGHT
PHASE 4: SPIRITUAL ELEVATION

Here is a summary of the preceding Life Management Plan. Sit down once a week and review the plan to see if you are addressing life management on *all* of its levels. Commit at least one hour a week to planning activities. Manage your life as if you were a chief executive. After all, your life *is* your business. And keep the journal or diary mentioned at the beginning of this plan. Write in it every day. Use binders with dividers—at least one divider for each level. Add your own levels and activities if you desire.

A Life Management Plan Outline
The Practical Level

TIME MANAGEMENT:
- ORGANIZE YOUR LIFE MANAGEMENT PLAN
- KEEP A SLEEP DIARY
  Regularity
  Adequacy
  Satisfaction
- KEEP A DAILY RECORD OF YOUR SCHEDULE FOR A MONTH
  Regularity
  Variety within the free time periods
  Adequacy in terms of health-promotion
  Utility in your addiction-affliction recovery process
  Satisfaction
- KEEP A RECORD OF HOW YOU SPEND YOUR FREE TIME
  Effects upon your recovery
  Pleasure derived
  Satisfaction
  Learning
- REMEMBER TO ALWAYS
  Plan ahead
  Have back up plans
  Do not change your schedule on the spur of the moment
  Build useful activities into your lifestyle on all levels

MONEY MANAGEMENT:
- KEEP A MONEY DIARY
  Sense of control
  Useful spending
- BUDGET

The Physical Level

EXERCISE MANAGEMENT:
- SEE YOUR DOCTOR
- KEEP A LIST OF ALL EXERCISE
- EVALUATE AND AMEND THIS LIST FOR:
  Regularity
  Adequacy
  Satisfaction

HYGIENE MANAGEMENT:
- TAKE A LOOK AT YOURSELF
- BUILD HYGIENE INTO YOUR SCHEDULE

The Nutritional Level

NUTRITIONAL MANAGEMENT:
- EAT REGULARLY
- EAT BALANCED
- EAT ENOUGH
- EAT NOTHING IN EXCESS
- EAT CALORIES WITH NUTRITIONAL VALUE

- KNOW WHAT YOU EAT. ASK YOURSELF:
  What did I eat and drink yesterday?
  What did I eat and drink each day of last week?
    for breakfast, if anything?
    for a morning snack?
    for lunch?
    during the afternoon?
    for dinner?
    for desert?
    for a midnight snack?
- ARRANGE THE ANSWERS TO THESE QUESTIONS INTO THE CATEGORIES LISTED IN THE FOOD CONSUMPTION CHART:
  MEAT, POULTRY AND FISH
  DAIRY PRODUCTS
  FRUITS and VEGETABLES
  NUTS and GRAINS
  EMPTY CALORIE FOODS
  SALT
  SUGAR
  CAFFEINE
  ALCOHOL
  OTHER DRUGS
  OTHER FOOD ADDITIVES
- KEEP A RECORD OF WHAT YOU EAT
- IMPROVE YOUR EATING BY EVALUATING YOUR EATING HABITS FOR:
  Regularity
  Balance
  Food Groups
  Water
  Empty Calorie Eating
  Satisfaction

The Chemical Level

CHEMICAL AND CRAVING MANAGEMENT:
- NOTE CRAVINGS
  Day
  Time
  Duration
  Object of craving
  How you respond to the cravings
  How you could respond differently to these cravings
- PLAN NEW RESPONSES

The Environmental Level

LIVING ENVIRONMENT MANAGEMENT:
- EVALUATE YOUR ENVIRONMENT FOR:
  Cleanliness
  Organization
  Attractiveness
  Comfort
- IMPROVE YOUR ENVIRONMENT ON A REGULAR BASIS

ENVIRONMENTAL TRIGGERS MANAGEMENT:
- IDENTIFY THE PHYSICAL TRIGGERS IN YOUR ENVIRONMENT
- WHEN NECESSARY, REMOVE THESE TRIGGERS

The Social Level

FAMILY LIFE MANAGEMENT:
- TIME MANAGEMENT
- MONEY MANAGEMENT
- NUTRITIONAL MANAGEMENT PLANNING
- OTHER MANAGEMENT AREAS RELEVANT TO THE FAMILY

WORK-LIFE MANAGEMENT:
- CONTROL WORK-RELATED TRIGGERS
- SUSTAIN WORK-LIFE WITHOUT BEING OVERCOME BY IT
- FIND SATISFACTION IN YOUR WORK

GENERAL SOCIAL LIFE MANAGEMENT:
- AVOID OR RISE ABOVE SOCIAL OR PEER PRESSURE
- GENERATE POSITIVE SOCIAL CONTACT
- FIND SOCIAL SUPPORT
- ENJOY HEALTHY SOCIAL TIME

The Psychological Level

EMOTION MANAGEMENT:
- FEEL AND FULLY EXPRESS THE PAIN AND JOY
- GIVE FULL VOICE TO FEELINGS
  Talk to friends
  Use taperecorder or video
  Write a diary
  See counselor or therapist

COMMITMENT MANAGEMENT:
- DECIDE TO BE COMMITTED
- FEEL COMMITTED
- FEEL COMMITTED ON ALL LEVELS

STRESS MANAGEMENT:
- KNOW STRESS
- RECOGNIZE STRESS AS OPPORTUNITY
  Remember that life can be stressful
  Identify stressful events in your individual and family history
  Stay current with your feelings
  Identify stressors as they appear
  When you identify a stressor or a symptom of stress, take measures:
    - Focus on the physical symptoms, whether they be faint or profound.
    - Concentrate on your breathing.
    - Do some physical exercise or stretching, if you can.
    - Call a friend.
  Always remember that life is stressful at every TURNING point
  Remember the opportunities that stress provides

The Energetic Level

PATTERN RECOGNITION MANAGEMENT:
- WEEKLY TRIGGER CHARTING

PATTERN REPAIR MANAGEMENT:
- REGULAR IN-SIGHT EXERCISES

The Spiritual Level

CONDITION MANAGEMENT:
- COMMITMENT
- ATTENTION
- FORTITUDE
- FAITH

PHASE MANAGEMENT:
- PHASE 1: STRUGGLE
- PHASE 2: PARADOX
- PHASE 3: INSIGHT
- PHASE 4: SPIRITUAL ELEVATION

Part IV

Insight

Knowledge is power.

—Old Adage

11

Insight Imagery: Seeing Inside Yourself

Many addicted individuals report that their urges or cravings for the object or objects of their addictions are overwhelming. If you are addicted, you may feel that you lose control during your cravings, and that your addictions commandeer your will power. What you must learn is that it *is possible to live through your cravings without responding to them addictively.* But, in order to learn how to do this, you must learn to face your cravings head on. Sometimes fear of the power of an urge or craving leads people to try to avoid constructive concentration on that urge or craving. This is a mistake. In this chapter, I suggest one method of looking urges and cravings in the eye. This method is an example of what I call *insight imagery.* I provide an exercise to demonstrate how insight imagery can help you to identify, confront, pay attention to, and ultimately live through your urges and cravings. In Chapter 12, I continue with this insight imagery, moving from work with more explicit images to work on the very subtle energetic level where we are forming implicit images and where they are forming our lives.

Imagery techniques are tools of focus. Memory imagery involves the visualization of memories. Visual imagery involves using the mind to see what is going on inside your body. Individuals who practice visualization can learn to direct increasing levels of concentration to special locations or conditions in their brains and bodies. By doing this, the *psyche* reaches into the *soma*, the mind reaches into the body, consciously and with a purpose. The individual who practices visual imagery thus achieves a greater degree of conscious control over his or her mental and physical health.

In the treatment of a particular health problem, whether that problem is biological or behavioral (the two are often related), imagery techniques can be tailored to the specific problem being addressed. Visual imagery is a process that reveals how the body and mind are related to each other. The first step in the healing process is to "see" the problem—to go inside the mind and body and take a good look at what's wrong. When the health problem is distinctly physical, this step is relatively easy. For example, a man suffering from cancer can be helped to "see" what is happening in his body by showing him slides of white cells attacking cancer cells, and x-rays showing the location and shape of the growths in his body.

Visualizing is not always this straightforward. It is one thing to form a rather accurate mental image of a tumor after looking at x-rays; it is another to "see" the energy patterns that may have caused that cancerous growth. And something like drug addiction proves still more difficult. In addition to the fact that all energy patterns affecting one's health are subtle and invisible, drug addictions have no one physical location to which they can be linked. There are no growths in the body to x-ray. White cells are not attacking a tumor. The experience of craving drugs, while extremely powerful, is not as concrete as are primary physical ailments. For drug-addicted persons to bring this experience into focus, they must learn to ask themselves: What is actually craving alcohol or drugs? What parts of my body are feeling this craving? How does this part of my body feel? Exactly where is this part of my body? What is its shape? Its size? Its temperature? Can a color be attributed to this temperature or texture? Can a color or set of colors be assigned to this part of the body and its feeling?

Whatever pattern addiction we are examining, we must keep in mind that many messages from our bodies go unnoticed. Learning to answer the questions listed above can teach you to focus on—to pay attention to—what you are actually feeling. These questions about the location, size, shape, temperature, texture, and color of your feelings can be answered by attaining a meditative state in which your concentration is focused so precisely that these characteristics are *seen*—known, understood—in your mind's eye. This is one technique of visual imagery. Another technique is to use your imagination to assign physical characteristics to your feelings. This method may seem arbitrary compared to the technique of directing your inner meditative vision, but imagination also leads to understanding. Where the focused imagination leads, concentration will follow. Whenever you feel that you cannot get actual information in the form of images from your body, use your imagination and make something up. (Note that the word *image* is contained in the word *imagination.*)

Individuals experiencing addiction picture their addictions in a myriad of ways. Every visualization that you *see* is an important piece of information about what is going on inside the psyche and the soma. Once the addiction has been visualized, the image can be changed—reduced, rearranged, manipulated, destroyed, or replaced with a more desirable picture.

This is done by first visualizing the craving and then creating a tool with which to resculpt or operate on the image of pattern addiction. Among the tools that have been created by people who use this technique are beams of light resembling lasers, balls of light that work like explosive bombs or absorbent sponges, chains or ropes that tie up the addictive image, knives or saws that cut it, paint brushes or crayons that redraw it, and hands that reach into it and operate on it. I like to use luminous soap suds that give off beautiful light.

With practice, this confrontation with the feeling of craving can be achieved each time you experience a craving. As a result, addiction can be clearly pictured and then operated on. In so doing, you can gain control over even the most powerful craving.

Visual imagery focuses your concentration on the experience of addiction in a way that allows you to be in command of your addictive behavior rather than subservient to it. Sometimes, when your addiction is explained in words, the problem seems intractable. But freedom from the confines of verbal thought brings power over addiction. The multitude of unknowns that overwhelm you are encapsulated in a single picture, a picture free of words, names, or labels. Imagery reduces complicated words to simple, powerful pictures.

I have included here an insight imagery exercise I did over a period of two decades with over 1,500 people addicted to drugs, alcohol, food, and other "things." Each time I did the exercise with a group of people, I explained that we would call whatever it was that each person was addicted to a "drug." This allowed people in the groups to understand their connections to the drug- and alcohol-addicted people in the groups and to see that the object of their addictions had become a drug for them. For example, chocolate cake means very little to me, but one gentleman I worked with simply could not stay away from it and would drive miles in the middle of the night to buy it. He was seriously overweight and felt he could not quit the cake. For him, chocolate cake was as addictive as heroin.

In order to do the exercise below, you will need a peaceful, quiet place where you will be comfortable and will not be disturbed. You will also need paper, a set of colored markers, and a tape player. If you are working on an eating habit or other explicit but nondrug addiction, just adapt this exercise to your own addiction. If you are working on an implicit addiction, try to find a drug or food you do crave sometimes. After you practice the exercise on this explicit craving, you can adapt it to the more implicit patterns you seek to transcend. Rewrite my exercise to suit your needs.

Record the following exercise on your tape recorder. Or have a friend record his or her voice. This exercise should be read very slowly in a very steady, calm voice. You or your friend may want to read the exercise over several times before recording. Once you have a recording and you are all ready, go ahead and play it. It helps to sit in darkened room. Now *relax, listen,* and *concentrate on these words.*

BASIC INSIGHT IMAGERY EXERCISE

Make yourself comfortable. Sit or lie in a comfortable position. If your legs are crossed or bent and you think you will begin to get cramps in your legs, stretch them out now. Find a position that you can be relaxed in for a long period of time.

Close your eyes. Breathe slowly. Try to stay awake but do not be concerned about dozing off or tuning out. If you do doze off, pay attention to where you start drifting. It is helpful to see where in this exercise you might tune out, if you do.

Now, think back to one of the last times that you succumbed to your addictive pattern.

We will begin now. When I ask a question, answer *only* that question. Do not answer out loud. Think *without words*. Think *in pictures* in your mind. Try to *see* the answer. Where you cannot see it, hear or taste or smell or feel the answer. When you have no answer, remember to *imagine* — just make up, invent an answer. *Imagining* and *imaging* are very close processes and each can supplement the other.

Again, think back to one of the last times you used your drug or did your habit. *Where* are you? Think only of the place where you were when you were last using your drug of choice or did your habit. Do not see yourself or anyone else in this place.

Imagine that you are a film maker. Take an invisible movie camera into your hands. You are making a film. It will be a slow motion movie. First you are setting the stage.... Look at the place where you were last doing your habit. Move the camera slowly around the room or the car or the building or the beach or wherever your place is. Remember to do this with your eyes closed, because you are looking at a place that is in your memory. Try to see the details: the colors of the walls, if there are walls; the colors that you would see around you; whether the place is messy or neat, orderly or chaotic. If you are indoors, what is hanging on the walls? What furniture is there? Try to feel and see in detail what the place is like. Sometimes your mind remembers details that do not easily come back to you when you consciously try to remember. There might be cracks in the wall, or ants in the corner, or spilled garbage somewhere. These things *are* there in your memory bank. The more relaxed you are, the more of these little pieces of the whole picture, the more bits of information, you will see. Remember, there are no people on your stage yet. And, remember, everything is in slow motion.

Now, the next assignment for you, the film maker, is to set the time of day. You may have to go back and look through the camera at the sky to see the time of day, or maybe you will look through the window or at the clock on wall. Show yourself what time of day it is. If you cannot remember, just pick a time. (By the way, if you haven't found a place yet, just *make up* a place. Pick a place. Remember, one of the rules of this game is that it is *okay* to use your imagination. Any time you don't have a memory or an image with which to answer a question, use something imaginary.)

So now you know the time of day. What is the air temperature? Are you warm or cold or neutral? If you are outside, do you know what the weather is like? If you are inside, what weather do you see through the window?

Now you will start adding people, if there are people, to this scene. See them arrive at this place. Are you a *lone user* — do you perform your habit alone? If so, you will not add people, not even yourself yet. Remember, you are *not doing* whatever your habit is at this point.

Now, if there are people in this place, turn your movie camera on each of these people and get some close-up looks at their faces. This may be the first time you have ever really looked at some of them. Try to see what these people look like. If there is just one person, get a close look at that one person's face. Look closely at the people. See what they are wearing, how they walk, how they sit, how their faces look.

Now it is time to look at *yourself*. Look at yourself more closely than you have ever looked before. You may have to pull the camera up to the ceiling and look down on yourself to see how you looked during the last time, or one of the last times, you gave in to your habit. You are not yet doing your habit, using your alcohol or drugs, or eating your habit foods, or doing whatever it is you are addicted to doing, but you *are* getting in touch with the state or states of mind, your feelings, your emotions, that you were in the last time you did so. Maybe you are partying, celebrating something wonderful that has happened. Maybe you are bored. Maybe you are having other feelings.

It is difficult to film states of mind. But use your movie camera. You are the star of your movie. See your face revealing your state or states of mind. Remember, there are all kinds of possible states of mind and many of them can be felt at the same time. Let yourself look through your camera lens at those states of mind that you are experiencing. If you *cannot* remember your states of mind, just *make them up*. If you like, try some states of mind on for size, just to see how they feel: While your eyes are closed, make faces showing different states of mind — a happy face, an irritated face, a sad face, a bored face, a tired face. Whatever expression reveals the state of mind you were in the last time you did your habit, see that expression in this exercise.

Now, in your slow motion movie, step back and look around the room. The people are there. You are there. You know what kind of day it is. You know what the place looks like. You know how you look. I want you to find some kind of flat surface — a counter, a tabletop, a chair. If you are in a car, maybe the surface is your lap, maybe it is the seat next to you. Maybe you are outdoors. I want you to find a flat surface in this place and turn your camera to that flat surface. If you do not have one, create a flat surface — some kind of place to put things down onto — and put that surface into your movie. If you still cannot think of a flat surface I will give you a table. Put a table into your room or place.

Now that you have a surface, take your camera and get ready to do some close-up shots. The things that are going to be on this flat surface are the objects, the paraphernalia, the things, that you associate with your habit. I want you to let these things appear very slowly. For some people, among these things might be a box of cigarettes and matches. For others, there will be a razor blade, a mirror and a sifter. For others there might be a bottle of scotch, a glass, and a bucket of ice. Maybe somebody has a combination of seemingly unrelated things, such as baking soda, a pack of cigarettes, and a beer to drink. Food addicts may have an array of foods or a few favorite foods on the table. Workaholics may have stacks of work and four or five telephones. Maybe there are all kinds of other objects and drugs out on this table. Remember whatever thing or activity or whoever you are addicted to is a called *your drug* in this movie. Remember that it is all right to make something up, to put anything you want on your table. This is your movie. You do not have to explain (to yourself or anyone else) why something (or someone) appears on (or at) your table.

When you see objects or drugs that are involved in your habit, take your camera and get a close-up shot of them. Do not touch any of these things with your hands; just take your camera and let your eyes look at them closely. *See the details.*

While you are doing this, a hand that you do not recognize reaches into this picture, into *your* movie, and starts putting more of these same things on the table, *more* than you have put there. Slowly the hand puts more and more things out. The table becomes very full. You see more and more of your drug objects, more and more of your paraphernalia and other things that you associate with your addiction. The table is getting so full that the stuff is spilling off of it. You're still filming it very closely, getting the close-up view, a microscopic view if you wish. You may be seeing marijuana leaves. You may be seeing the ice cubes or bubbles in some drink. You may be seeing food, crumb by crumb....

You are seeing a variety of objects of your choice. You are looking *very closely* at these things now. As you look closely, you, the film-maker, begin to realize that you are *connected* with this stuff. You have had a lot of experiences using this stuff. Your mind and your body remember using this stuff. And somehow now the camera falls away from or dissolves out of your hands. You find your hands becoming very stiff. Now put your stiff hands out in front of you, with your eyes closed. Stretch your fingers out. Again, be sure your hands are very stiff. Reach out, but do not take into your body or self any of the objects of your addiction. Do not actually use anything on your table. Just reach out stiffly and touch all the stuff on the table in front of you.

Feel these objects. Let your hands be stiff while you do this, so that you are putting some stress into your efforts. Your hands are feeling the stress of your relationship to these objects — cigarettes or drinks or drugs or food or whatever they may be. Now you find yourself preparing this stuff for your use. You are not actually using it yet, just preparing it. You are cutting, pouring, sifting, stirring, mixing, piling, organizing, opening some packages — whatever you need to do to prepare to use your so-called drug objects.

Let your hands act out the necessary motions. Remember to keep your eyes closed while you do this project. Let yourself act it out. If you are preparing to smoke a cigarette, imagine that you shake the package, pull one out, put the cigarette to your lips, light the match, but please do not light the cigarette. If you are preparing to smoke a marijuana cigarette, imagine yourself pulling out a rolling paper, shaking some leaves onto the paper, carefully rolling the cigarette, licking the gum, sealing the paper, twisting the ends. Put the cigarette in your mouth, but do not light it. If you are getting ready to snort a line of coke, cut up a line, roll a bill, get yourself all ready, but please do not snort it. Similarly, you may pour yourself a drink, drop in some ice, mix in whatever you like, but do not drink it. Just act out the feeling of preparing or getting ready to do whatever it is that your addiction drives you to do. Over and over again, go through the motions of getting ready to do your habit. You can adapt this to any explicit pattern addiction.

Now you begin to feel a little more tension. And you begin to feel tension in more than just your hands. You feel tense, because this is a tense experience. Many people think of acting out their habits as being relaxing. But there is a tension to habits, and often we do not get in touch with that tension.

Now I want you to let your hands and your arms and your shoulders become very tight. I want you to imagine that you are moving your drug, whatever that may be, and any related paraphernalia that you are using, toward your body, as if you were about to use the substance. You are moving it toward your mouth, nose, or vein. As you find yourself *getting ready* to use it, you also find yourself getting very tense. Your body tenses up all over. You may be having a lot of other reactions, too. You feel a great deal of *tension!* Still you move it closer, closer, closer, closer to your body.

At this moment I want you to *freeze. Freeze* your movie. *Freeze* this room with your eyes closed. *Stop time.*

Now that time is stopped, ask yourself what are you *feeling most* in *your body right now*. You may feel something, or you may not consciously feel anything. I will give you some examples of what you may be feeling. If you are not consciously feeling anything, you may want to pick one these feelings and imagine you are feeling it: excess salivation, watery mouth, pain or sensation in the sinuses, throbbing head, headache, cold or hot rushes, cold or hot patches, numb patches around the body, a feeling of excitement in your throat, a burning in the chest, a knot in the stomach, a tightness in your legs, lead in your feet, sexual excitement. There are so many things you may be feeling. Most of the time we miss these feelings because we are so hooked into our habits; we run on automatic. We are not in touch with what we are feeling. This time, you concentrate on what you are feeling. Pick one or two of these feelings and let yourself *feel*. Invent a feeling if you do not have one.

Now identify the part or parts of your body that you are most aware of right now. You are definitely aware of something. It may just be the feeling of touching the chair or the floor. But it may be a feeling that has come out of your experience or one of the feelings that I just mentioned. Now pretend that one of your fingers is a colored felt pen. Pick a color, and outline the area of your body that you are most aware of. Outline that part. If the area is hot, use a hot color. If it is cold, use a cool color. Now pretend to color this area in; you may want to use some other colors. If you have a knot in your stomach, draw the knot. If your heart is beating quickly, you may want to use some color that reminds you of a fast pulse, high blood pressure, and maybe tension. Everybody sees his or her own colors. You may be feeling other things in this part or some other part of your body. You may have been having feelings without knowing which part of the body those feelings are coming from. Try to give those feelings a place in your body.

Now that you have identified your feelings, imagine that you are washing your hands with some very sudsy soap. While your eyes are closed, put your hands in front of you and start washing yourself. Keep your eyes closed and feel yourself washing all over. Now you notice that the sudsy soap you are using is giving off light. It's giving off a beautiful, gleaming light. Touch your face and wash it with this amazing light. You will notice that your skin is becoming light, too; the soap is leaving light everywhere.

Now wash your neck. It feels really good to touch your skin. Wash your arms, spread this soap full of light all over your arms. And as you wash, massage your body. Imagine the feeling of being massaged by a penetrating light that leaves you glowing. Massage your chest and your torso. Be sure to reach down and massage your legs. You are washing yourself with healing light. As you massage and wash, you are breathing very slowly. Whenever you can, take a deep breath. . . .

Don't forget to wash your feet. Reach down and touch your feet with this sudsy, light soap. When you have done that, bring your hands back up, maybe to your shoulders or your upper arms — to some part of your body. Touch yourself somewhere and breathe deeply, very deeply and very slowly. Remember that, anytime you are feeling anxious or are feeling an urge to do your habit, you can live through this feeling. You can focus on it, go inside of it, give it a place in your body. You can work with this feeling. Your mind created it, and *you can change your mind*. . . .

Very good. You did a great job! Keep your eyes closed a littler longer. Now, ask yourself the following questions: If you fell asleep during the exercise, when did you fall asleep, during what part of the story? If you are sleeping now, how deeply are you sleeping? Can you hear me on some level? If you are awake, did you participate in the story? How did you feel about the story? And if you saw some images, what were those images? If you felt some feelings, what were those feelings? If you gave those feelings a place in your body, what place did you give them? Finally, when you washed yourself with the light, how did those images and feelings change? Where did they go? What happened to them? Now just lie there for a while and imagine that you are still giving off that beautiful light. Notice that simply causing your mind to focus on giving off light is a relaxing and healing process.

(Pause.)

Now stay with your eyes closed for a few minutes and do nothing but feel whatever you are feeling.

(Pause.)

In a few moments, open your eyes. Now, before you talk to anyone, draw what you saw or felt during this exercise. If you gave a feeling a particular place in your body, or if you saw a feeling as a particular shape or color (or shapes and colors), draw those places, shapes and colors. Draw anything else about this experience that you can remember. Please use no words at all in your drawing. Please do not speak until the drawing session is over.

Think in pictures.

END OF VISUAL IMAGERY EXERCISE

Well? How did it go? Take a look at your drawing. What do you think it is trying to tell you? What are *you* trying to tell you? You can learn to read your visual images like messages from deep inside you. Once you are able to see your images, you can change them in any way you like, or you can eliminate them. Take a look at the following pictures. They were all drawn by people doing this insight imagery exercise. Figures 11.1 through 11.10 were done by drug- (including alcohol and nicotine) addicted people in the early stages of recovery. Figures 11.11 through 11.15 were done by persons suffering from multiple explicit addictions. Figure 11.16 was done by a woman with an overeating problem. Figures 11.17 and 11.18 show more advanced and intricate insights into deeper, more implicit, levels of pattern addiction. You will see, in this collection, images similar to those you may have had during this exercise or at other times. Many images of cravings, longings, addictive sensations, psychological, emotional, energetic, and spiritual states are held in common among people and among addictions. It is as if a nonverbal mind language exists—one which says so much more than words and which has not yet been catalogued by man. We all have so much in common.

The following descriptions apply to the insight imagery drawings at the end of this chapter.

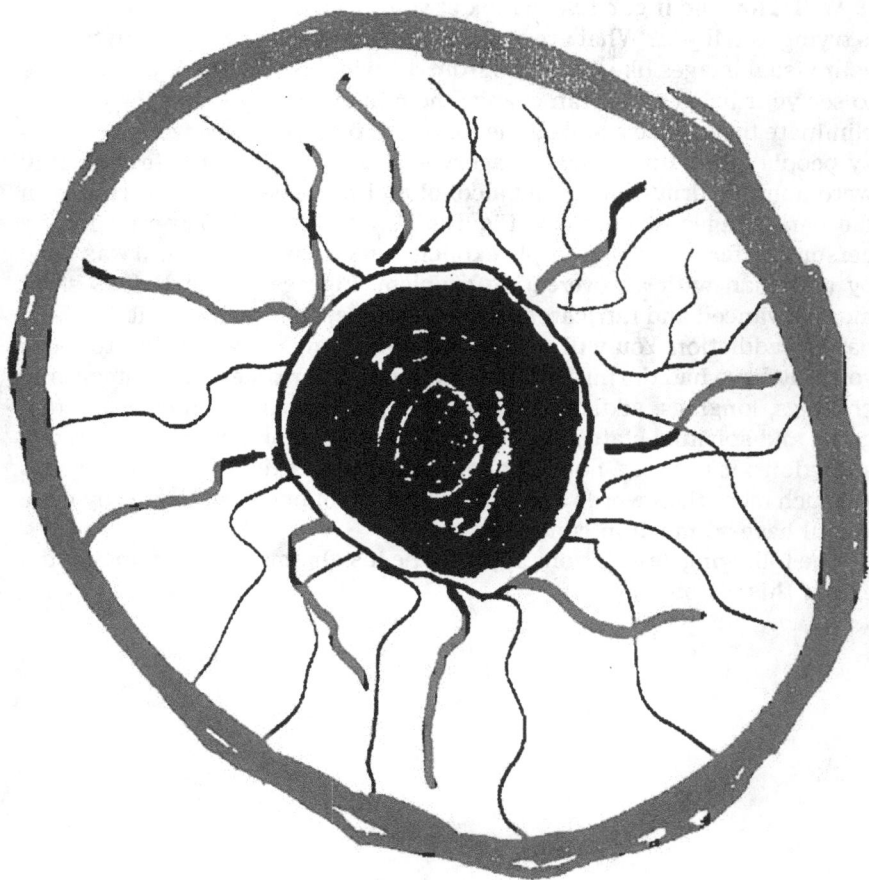

Figure 11.1: The center of pressure and craving was the eyeball for one individual. During a strong craving, he reported an irritation around his eyes along with a feeling of mesmerizing suction through his irises into the back of his head. Whenever the suction consumed him, he "gave in," and, against the directions given in the exercise, imagined himself using his drug of preference.

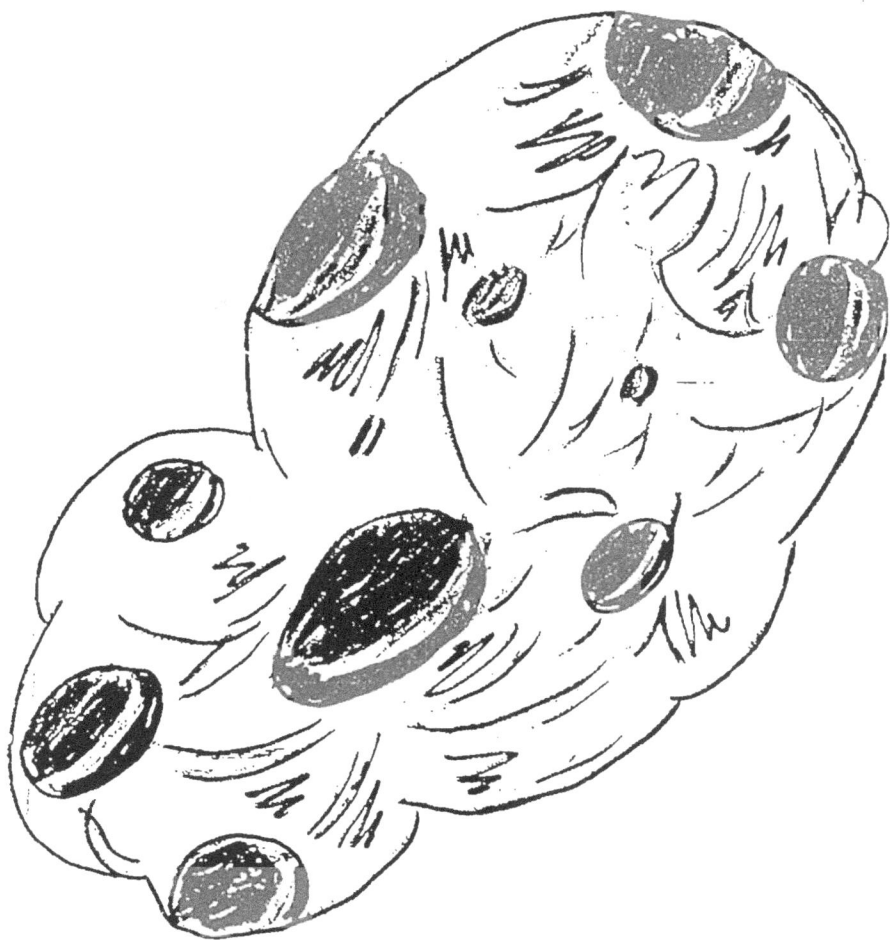

Figure 11.2: A second individual reported that, when he "went inside" he found his craving in his yellow-and-white-colored stomach, in the form of "black and blue globs." He later took a "laser beam" into this visual image and burned out (with a "clean, cool light") the heavy globs. This allowed him to experience control over this craving.

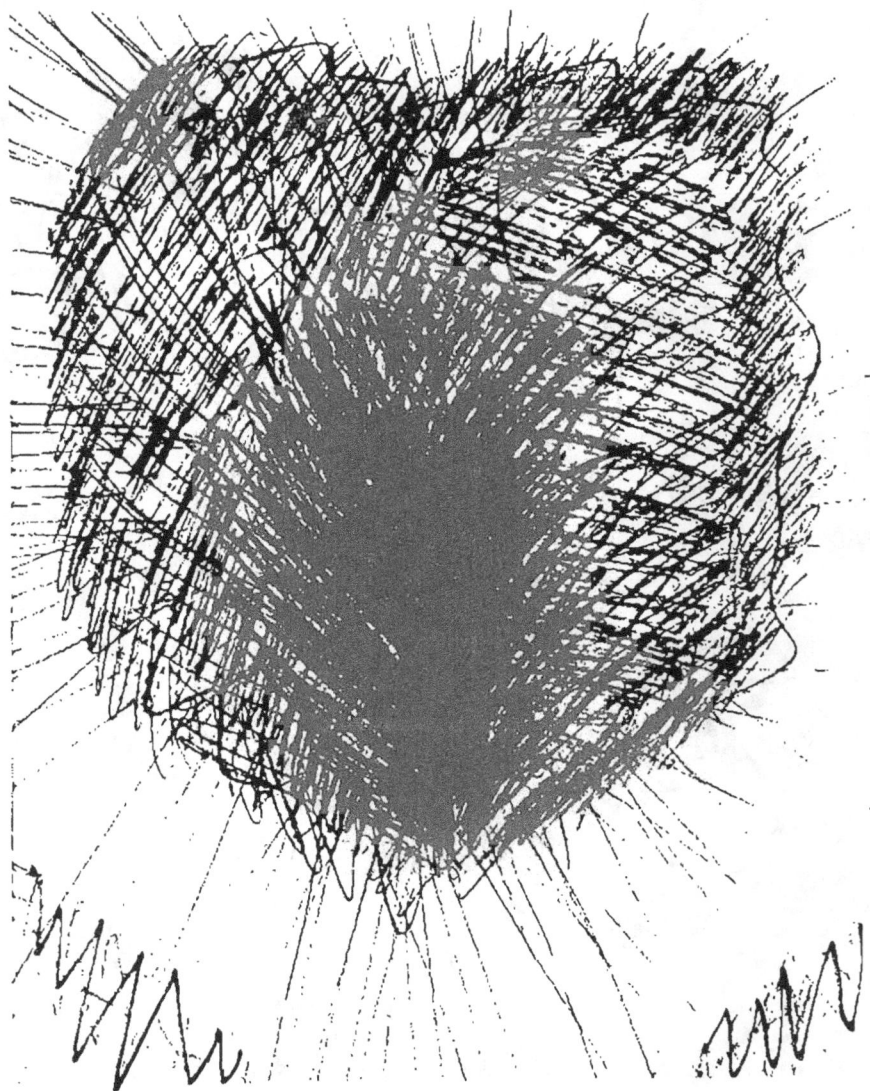

Figure 11.3: This is a drawing of a "fierce burning sensation" in the chest and "a pain in the windpipe" experienced by a coke (cocaine) smoker when feeling the urge to smoke his "base." In color, this picture is a fierce scribbled combination of red, yellow and black.

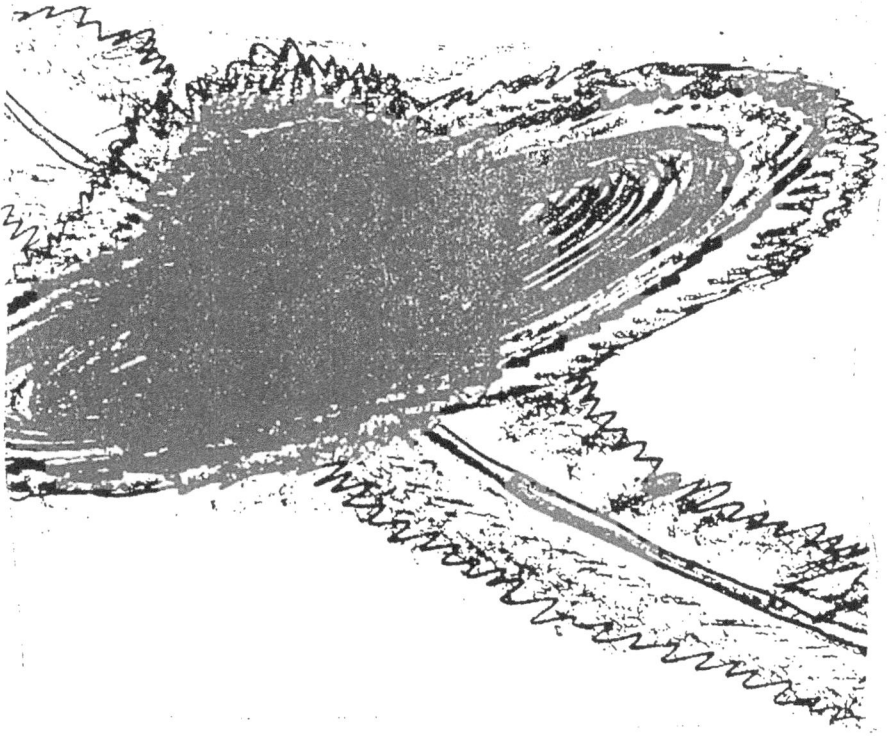

Figure 11.4: "Whenever I crave pot or coke or even a beer, a dark planet invades my brain," explained another addicted person. She later took a ball of blue light into the image to replace the dark planet, as if doing surgery on her universe.

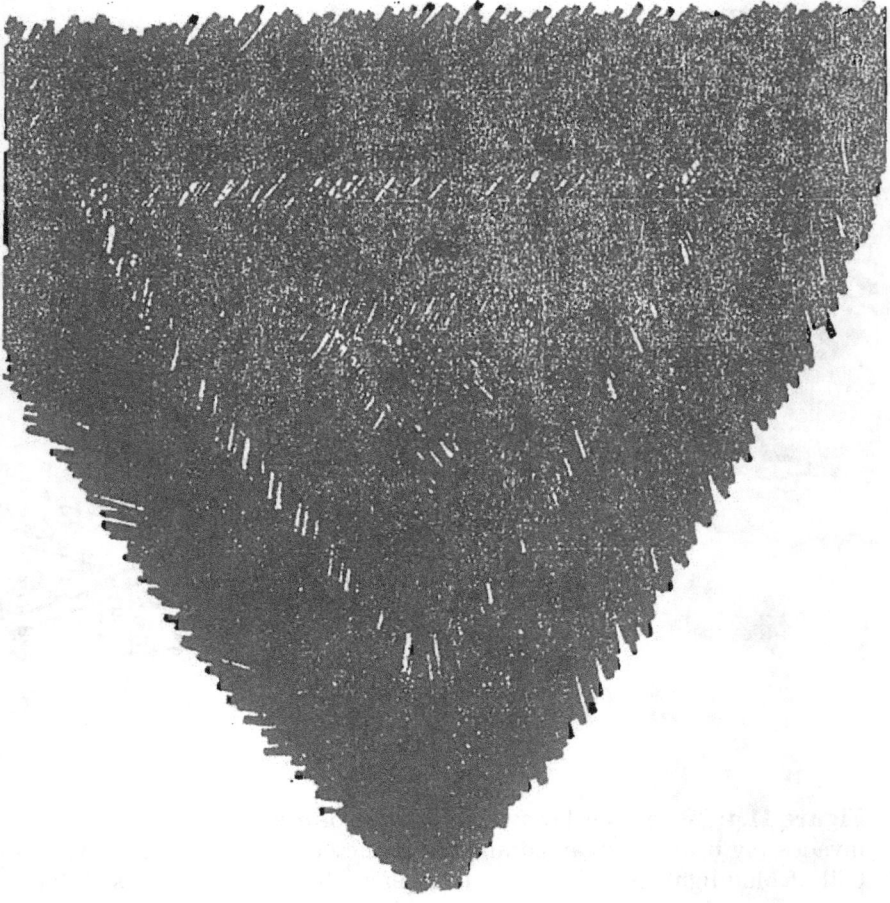

Figure 11.5: Once they learn "to go inside and see," many drug and food addicted persons report dense concentrations of craving encircled by perimeters of various colors. "The problem is that I keep being drawn into the center of this picture—the worst part, the black hole," reported the author of this figure. "It feels like there is no escape from that hole. I get there and I just give in to all my urges. For me, addiction is a vicious triangle which I live inside. I want to learn to feel like it is smaller than I am. Right now, it is so big to me that I am lost in it."

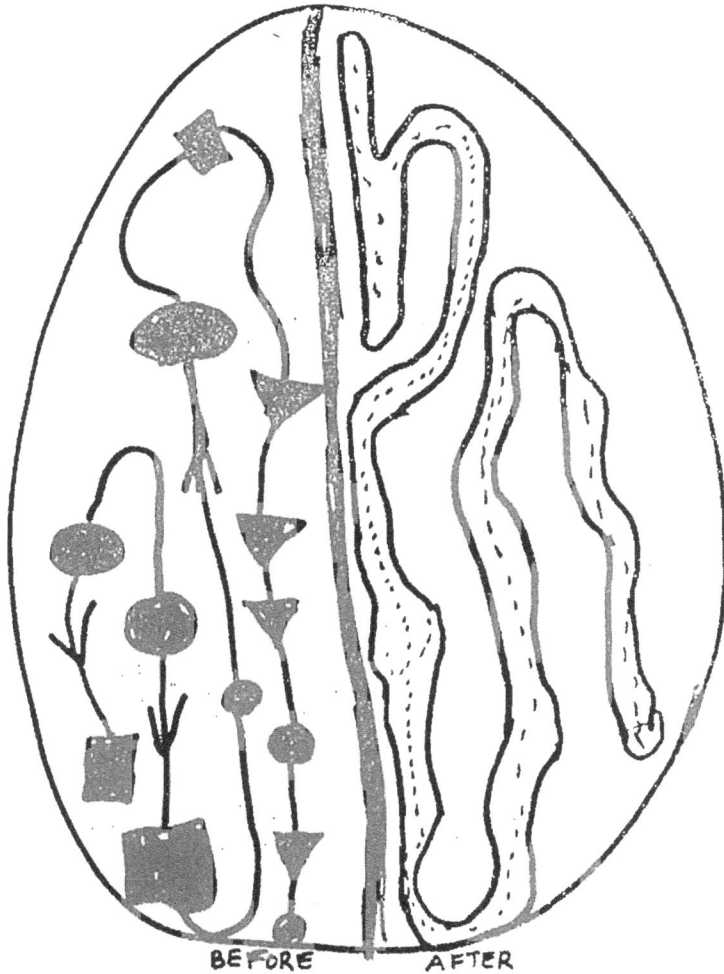

BEFORE   AFTER

Figure 11.6: "This is me before and after my drug use," explained another individual. First I feel all tense and blocked up, like I'm constipated all over (left side of the circle), and then I feel soothed when I satisfy my craving (right side of the circle)." This individual learned to clear out the knots and blocks in her visual image of craving by sending soothing hands into the image. In this way she was able to soothe her craving without using her drug. This sense of constipation as part of the urge to use is frequently expressed by cocaine and caffeine addicted persons.

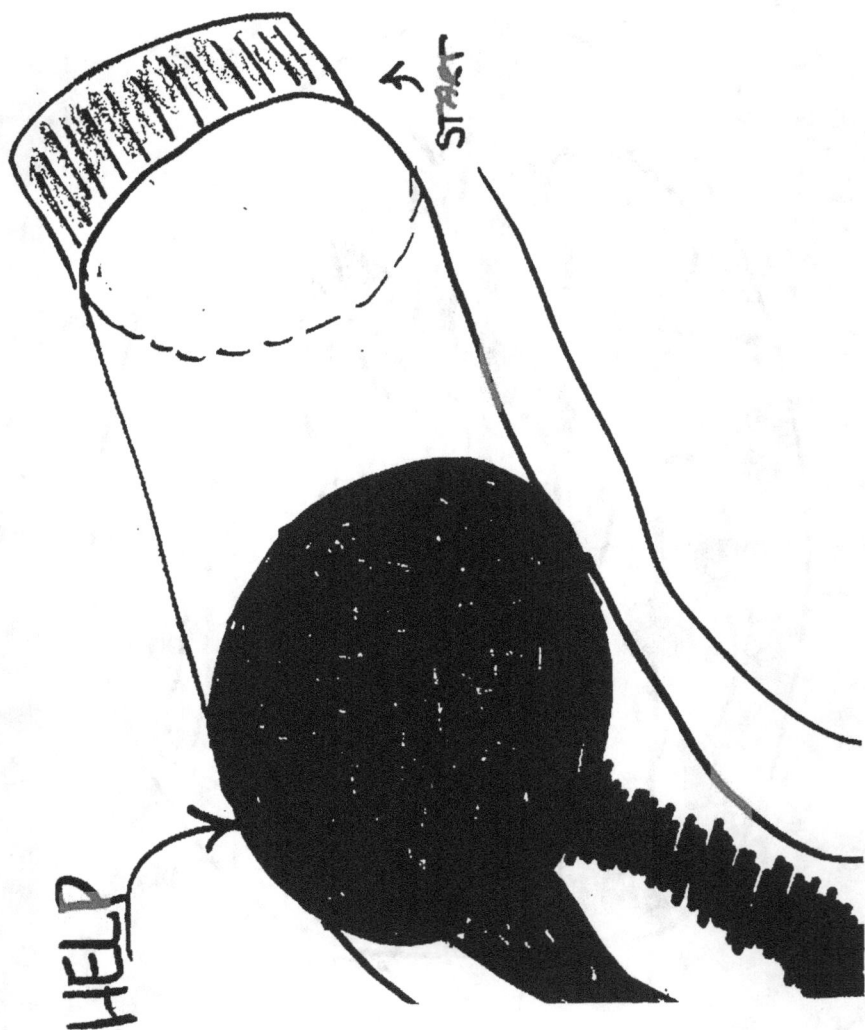

Figure 11.7: This is a cocaine smoker's picture of addiction. At the start, there is a pleasant and light sense of desire for the drug in the mouth. Then, deeper in the throat, there is a forceful darkness surrounding jagged pieces of intense red light. These pieces of red light are symbols of the power, the lure of the drug, for this individual. He taught himself to concentrate on relaxing his throat and reducing his craving by changing the colors in his throat to lighter, happier ones.

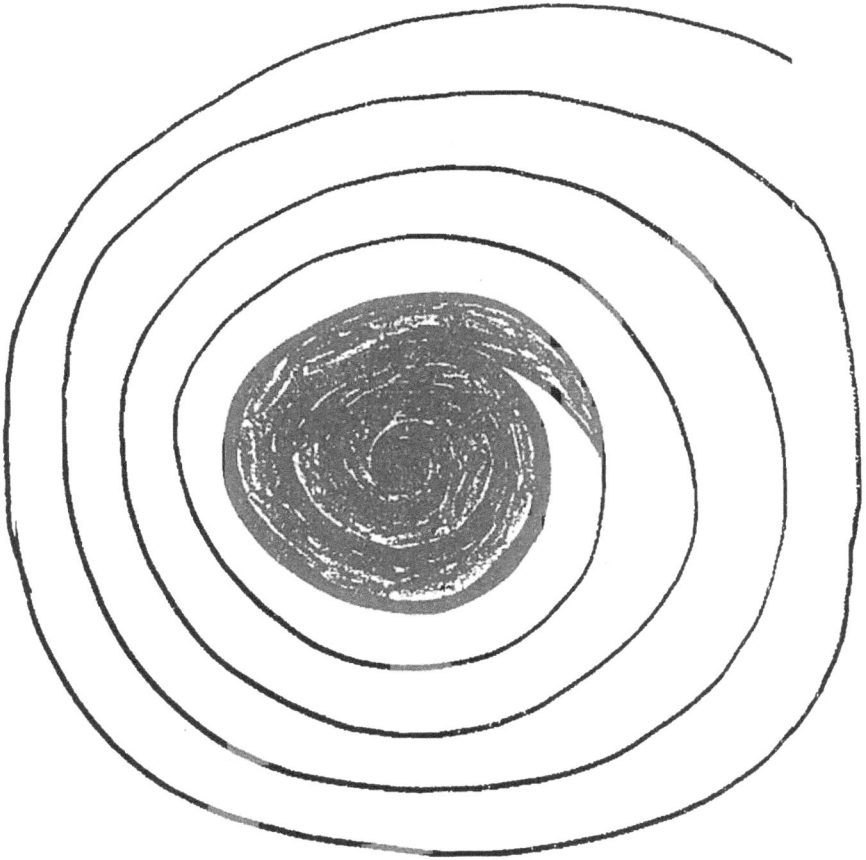

Figure 11.8: This image of irreversible, hypnotic suction into a black hole is common among the addicted persons. The object of one's addiction is seductive, compelling, and demanding. The fearful sense of powerlessness, of succumbing to the craving, is slowly absorbed by a magnetic mesmerism with the object of addiction.

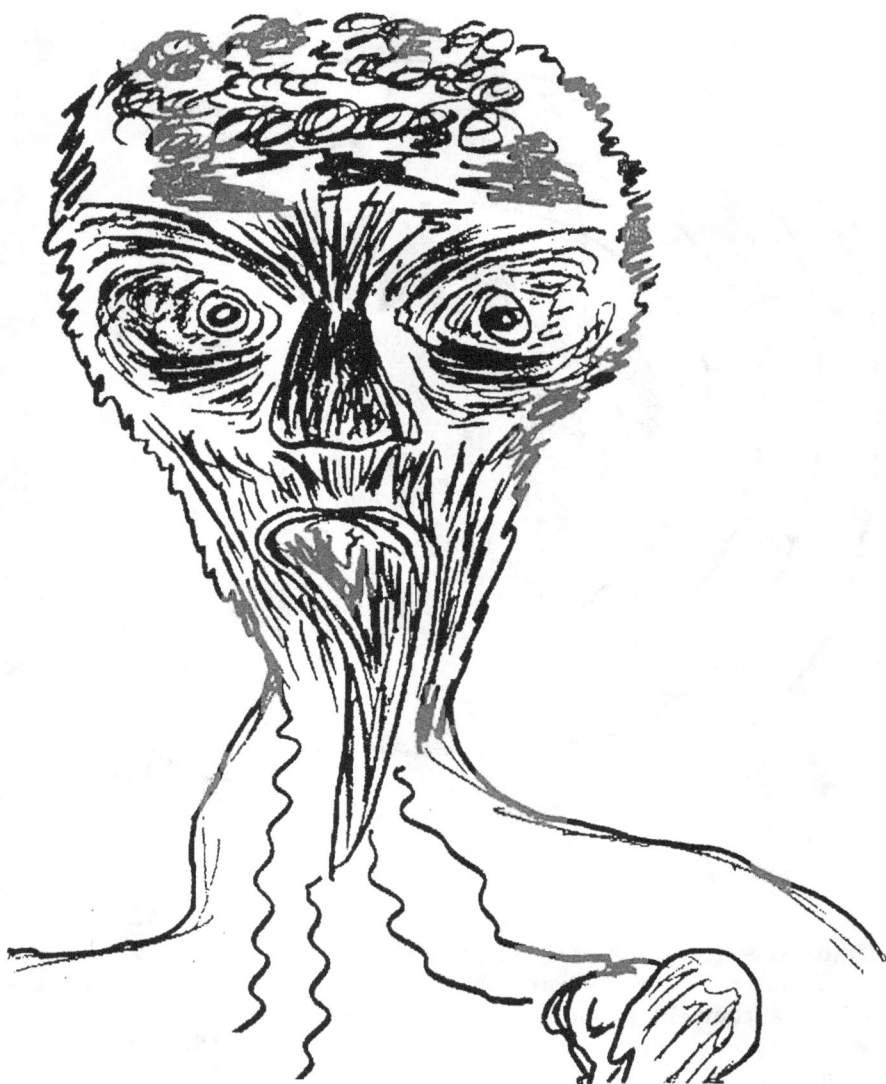

Figure 11.9: This is a self-portrait drawn by a person craving his three favorite drugs: marijuana, cocaine injected intravenously, and liquor. He had never done any drawing before. Witnesses were amazed at the resemblance between his drawing and his face.

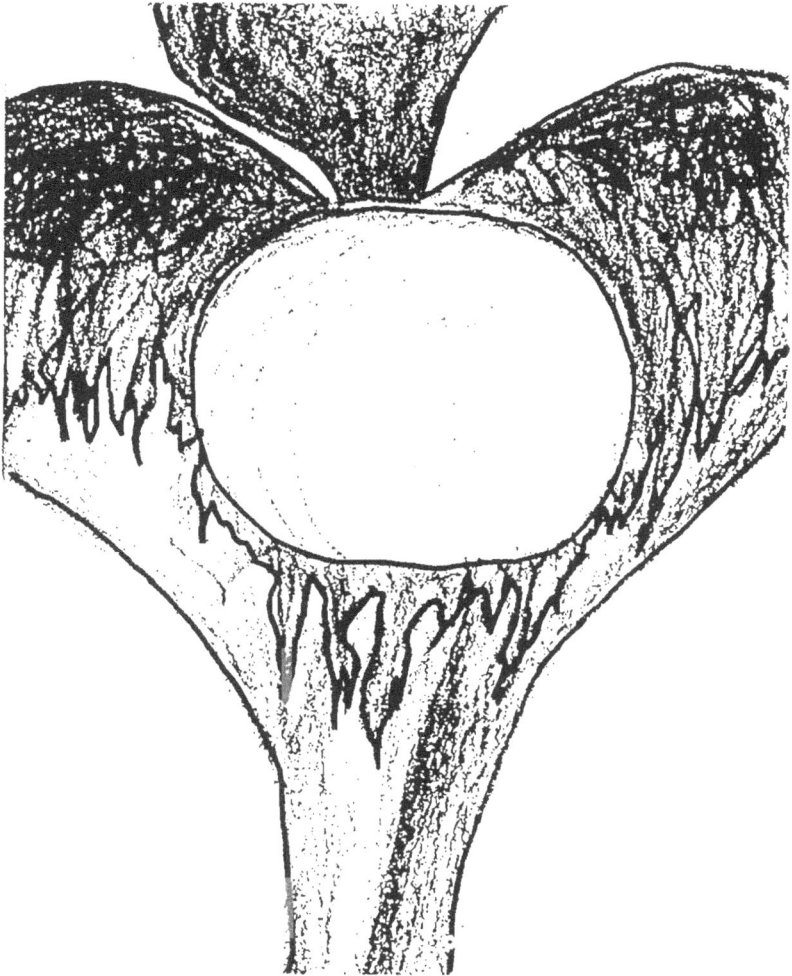

Figure 11.10: For some addicted persons, anticipated pleasure means that the picture of craving is somewhat pleasant. The addicted person who drew Figure 11.10 found his picture of addiction to be a glowing ball of yellow light in his chest. The rest of his body, where not touched by anticipation, was not in an equally positive state. He learned to expand this ball of yellow light into his extremities via visualization, without the aid of drugs. He learned that the mind can induce sensations as effectively, and even more effectively, than drugs.

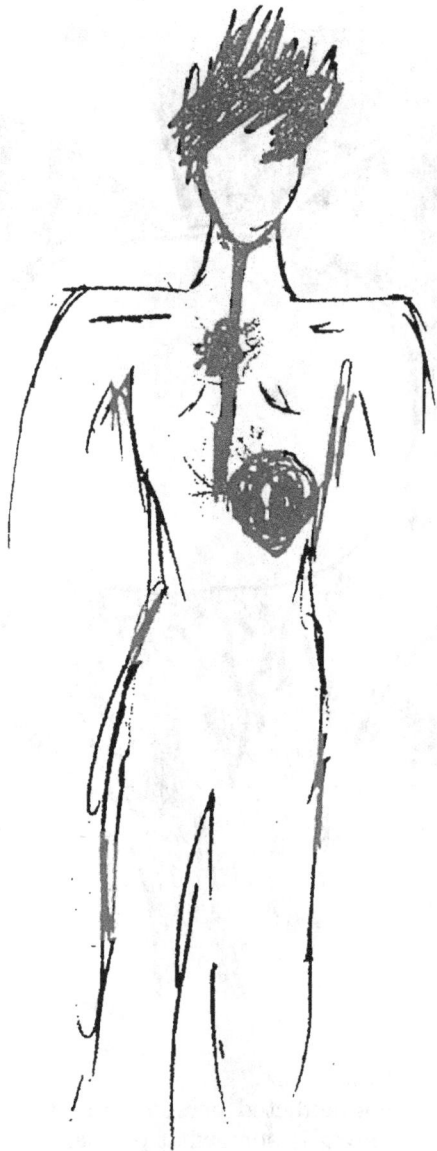

Figure 11.11.

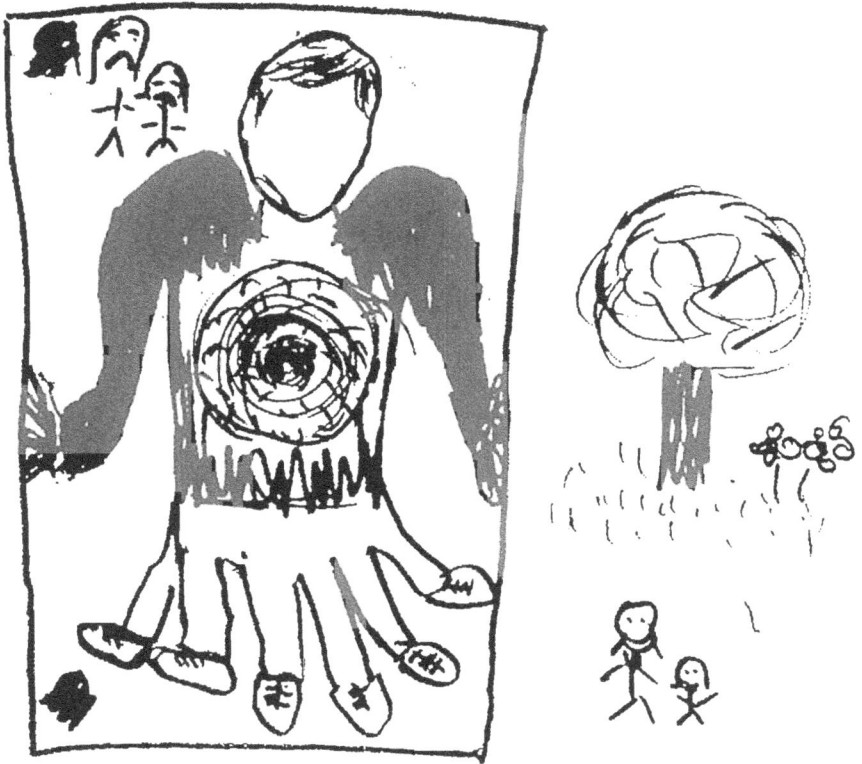

Figure 11.12.

Figures 11.1 through Figures 11.15: Many people who do this exercise visualize their entire bodies. Figures 11.11–11.15 were drawn by a group of individuals, each of whom was struggling with multiple addictions to drugs, foods, and compulsive behaviors. A sense or picture of the whole self is an excellent starting point for the process of increasing self-awareness. Sometimes detail of focus is sacrificed by focusing on the whole self. However, with training, detail can be developed as a next step.

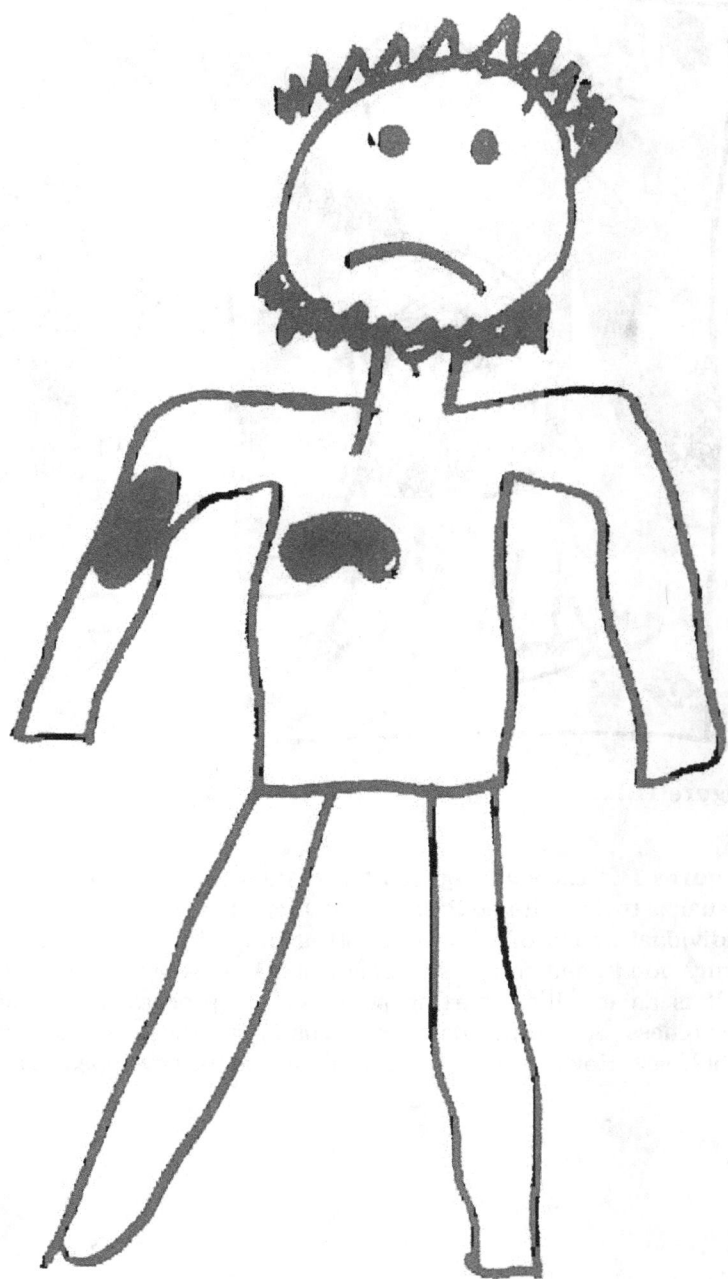

Figure 11.13.

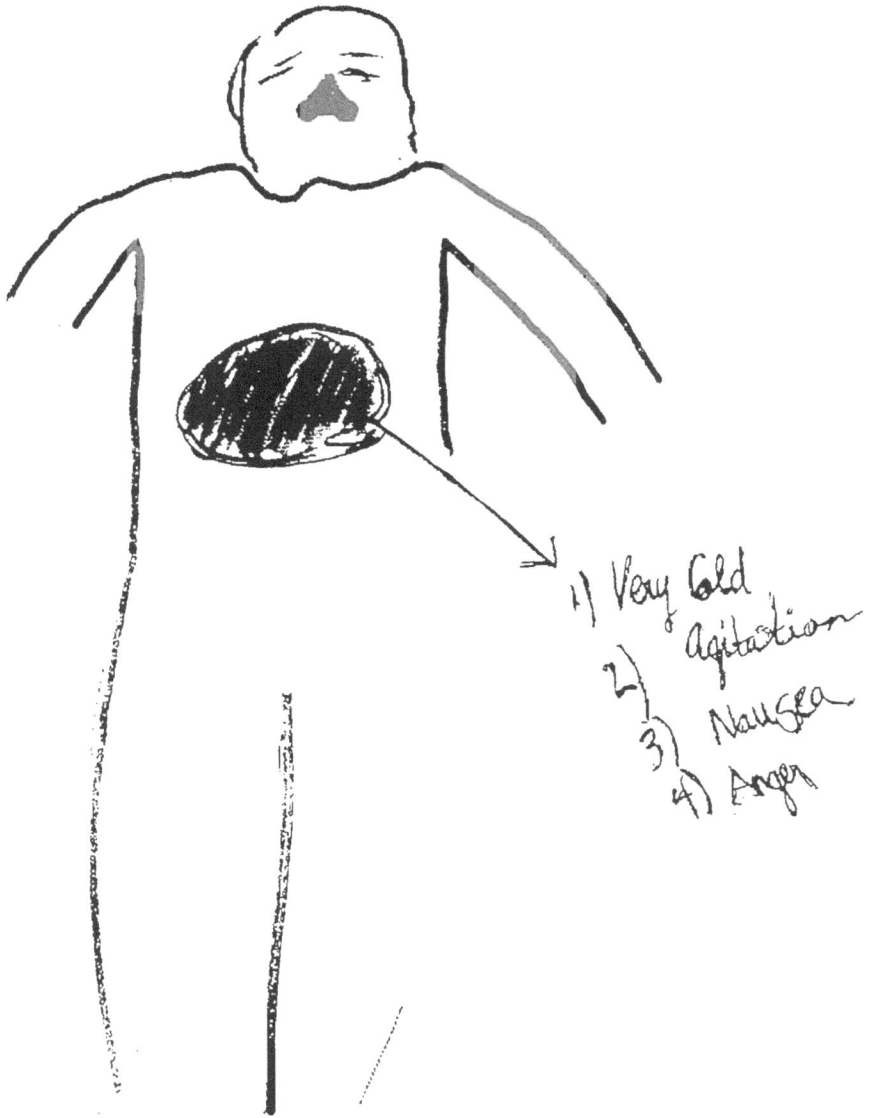

1) Very Cold
   Agitation
2)
3) Nausea
4) Anger

Figure 11.14.

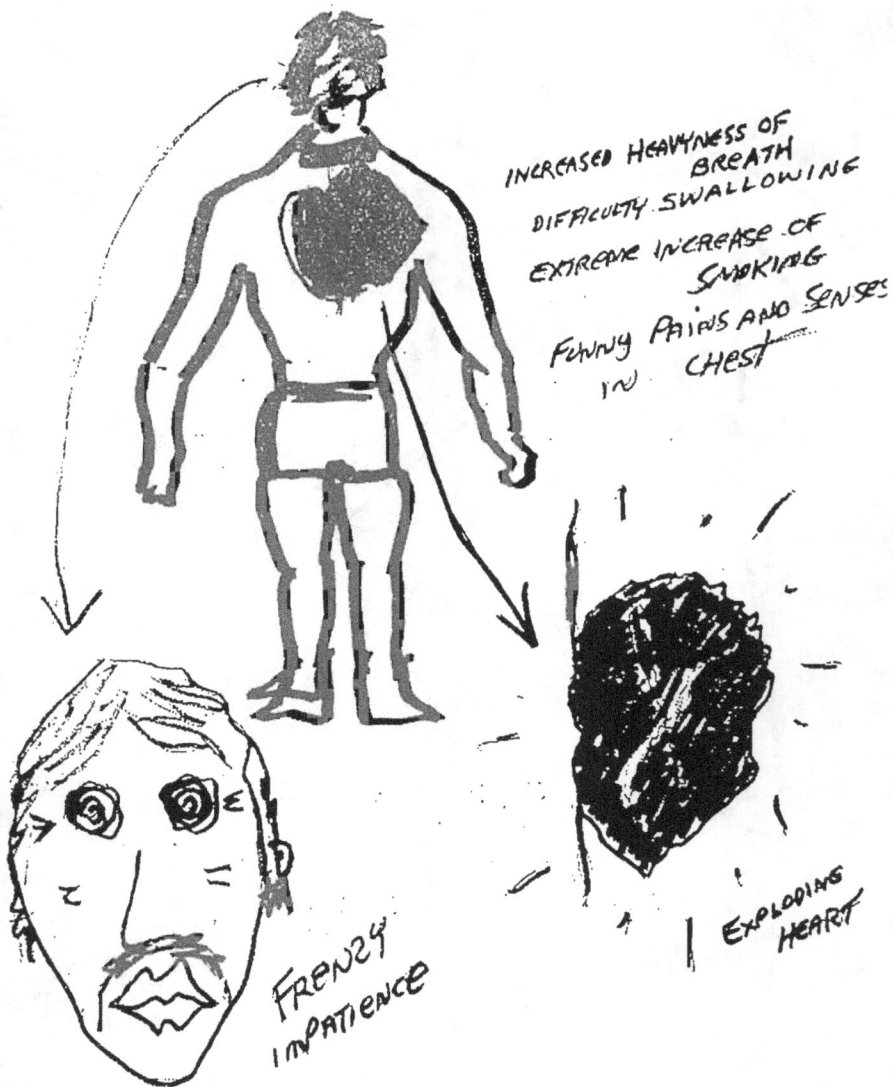

INCREASED HEAVYNESS OF BREATH

DIFFICULTY SWALLOWING

EXTREME INCREASE OF SMOKING

FUNNY PAINS AND SENSES IN CHEST

FRENZY IMPATIENCE

EXPLODING HEART

Figure 11.15.

128

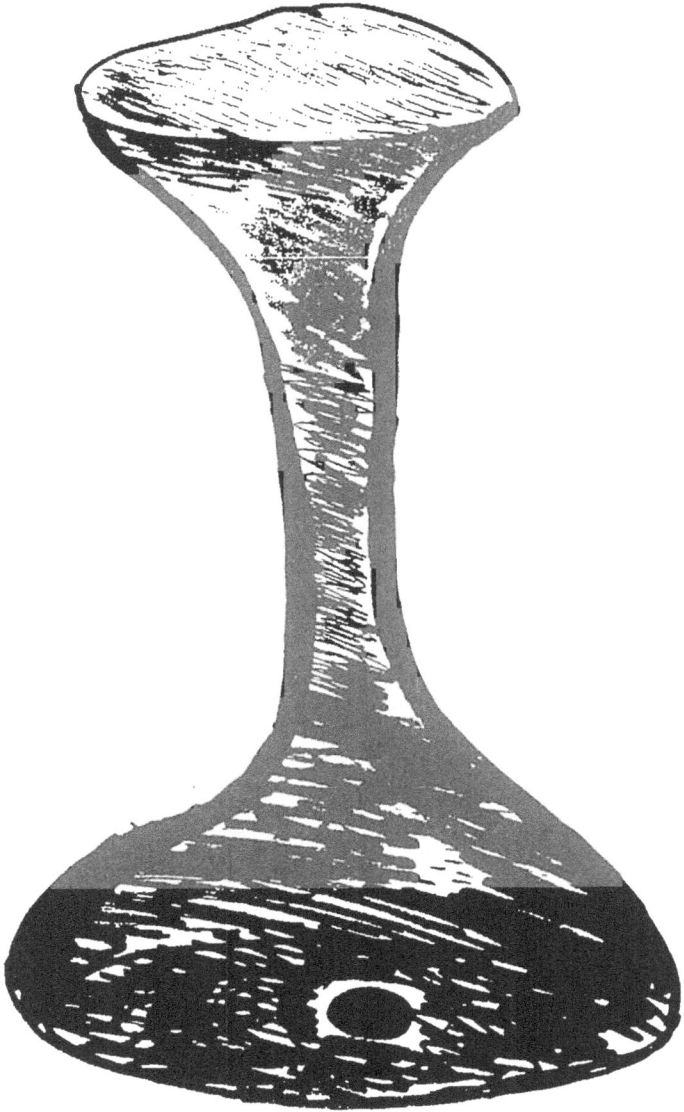

Figure 11.16: This is a drawing done by a overeater who was able to look closely at the mouth-to-esophagus-to-stomach connection. She found that the craving for oral gratification of eating looked and felt pleasurable in the mouth and culminated in a miserable black hole in the stomach.

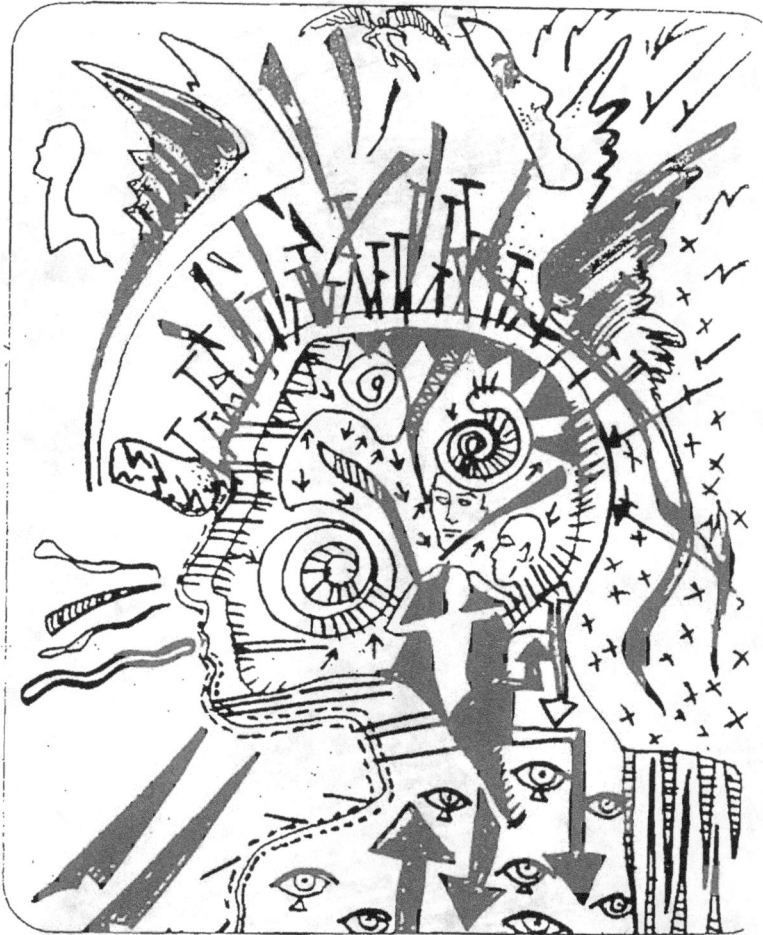

Figure 11.17.

The author of Figure 11.17 was looking at the implicit pattern addictions that had driven his explicit drug, food, sex, and mood-swing patterns addictions and chronic migraine headaches for two decades. During the exercise, he filled his table with the objects representing as many of his addictions as he could visualize. When he was told to freeze, this set of sensations and energies he depicts in his drawing became very clear in his mind. He later used his drawing to begin studying the flow and blockage of energy in his head and body. The exercise in Chapter 12 proved very helpful to him.

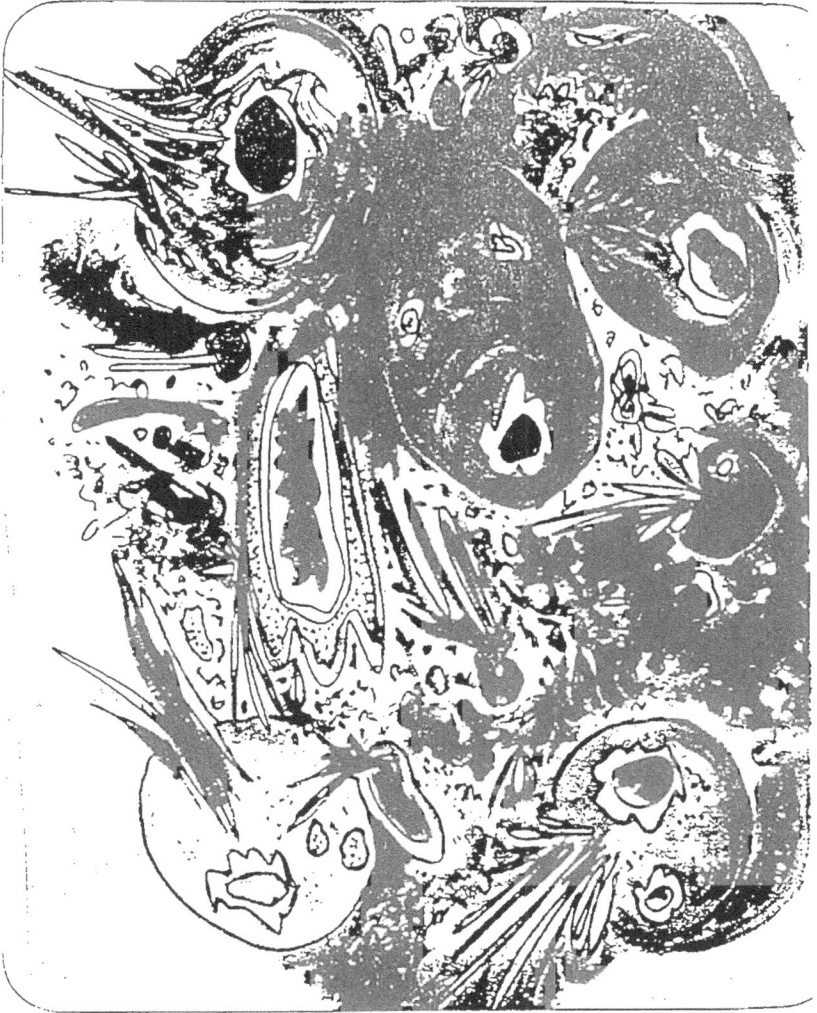

Figure 11.18.

In Figure 11.18, an insight regarding implicit energy pattern took place on what was described by the drawer as the "microbial" level. She felt that she became aware of a gnarled metropolis of cells, all competing for nourishment and stimulation and all manifesting competing demands. She felt that, right down to the cellular level of her organism, she was not unified with herself and that her energy was congested. I will say more about energy in Chapter 12.

12

Mindstyle Surgery

A lifestyle is a complex entity, something which, over time, takes on a form—a life—of its own. A lifestyle begins to develop at birth. Genetic influences on lifestyle, brought into the world through the baby's chromosomal composition, interact immediately with the baby's environment. (In fact, the genetic–environmental interaction actually begins in the womb.) At no time and in no way do genes and environment operate separately of each other. Each of us is a product of our genetic heritage (which is determined largely by ancient environmental pressures on the reproduction of our ancestors) and of the environments in which we live in our present lifetimes. We are born with both genetic preprogramming and the predisposition, a biological mandate, to acquire new programming: biotechnological robots with individualized personalities and accompanying individualized life experiences and lifestyles. Our minds have either been styled by a great godlike engineer, or by evolution, or, perhaps, by something similar to both.

Within the narrow parameters determined by our biological programming, we experience varying levels of free will. We make what seems to be a never-ending stream of personal choices. We consciously relegate some of our activities to our automation units—memorizing phone numbers and speeches and friends' birthdays. We also do this relegation to automatic on a subconscious basis, usually because it is expedient. We remember some phone numbers without trying. Many of us cannot even recall how we memorized our addresses or our social security and other identification numbers. We conveniently remember how to type, how to ride a bicycle, how to spell thousands of words, how to add, how to respond to a red traffic light, how to speak our native tongues.

Memorization is accomplished through repetition. Each time we do something, a series of biochemical-electrical signals, a set of bits of energy, races through our brains and nervous systems. The set of biochemical-electrical bits of energy, and its path through the body, can be memorized. The more we repeat an action or a thought or a feeling, the more ingrained in our memories it will be. I say action *or thought or feeling*, because it is not only actions that are transmitted via energy bits from the body and brain into the brain's memory bank, it is thoughts and feelings as well.

Responses to social and emotional events can become quite automatic. Every time Uncle Joe sees Uncle Dan, he starts to wheeze and swear. Every time Mark and Evelyn argue, Mark's blood pressure goes up. Every time little Chester hears his parents argue, he feels poorly about himself. Every time Dick and Norman get together at social events, they overeat. Every time Hal goes to a party, he drinks too much. Eventually, just the anticipation of the precipitating event triggers such a response. Now Uncle Joe starts to wheeze and swear two days before Uncle Dan arrives for his annual visit. Mark's blood pressure goes up as soon as he starts to think that Evelyn is in a bad mood. Little Chester feels poorly about himself most of the time now, as it seems to him that his parents are always fighting. Dick and Norman both overeat at social events similar to the ones where they meet. Now Hal drinks too much anytime he is around other people, whether or not they are partying. The memory of the precipitating social-emotional event has become a trigger for each of these people.

Some trigger memories are much more subtle than arguments or social events. Repeated exchanges of energy between individuals, or between individuals and their environments, are ingrained into the memories of all persons involved. For example, it becomes very difficult for a couple, even a couple who so desires, to break a thirty-year-old marital power structure. Perhaps the major decisions in the family are made by the biggest income earner and the most educated of the two spouses. If, twenty years into the marriage, the lower income-earning and less educated spouse earns an advanced degree and lands a high-paying job, that spouse may demand a shift. But both spouses may find that they slip back into the old pattern out of habit. All accompanying subservience and low self-esteem, stored over twenty years by the low-income-earning spouse, seems to linger, although that spouse feels that the reasons for these emotions are gone. And, the once higher income-earning spouse may continue to expect the other spouse's subservience, even though the (presumed) monetary justification for it is now gone.

Another example. A mother constantly undergoes rapid mood swings, which confuses her child throughout her childhood. But the child's confusion is never discussed and is not made explicit. Instead, the child feels continuously insecure about emotional states, especially happy ones. These happy times could change at a moment's notice, with no advance warning and no explanation. The child is always waiting for the other shoe to drop and always holding her breath. Finally when this child reaches her middle age, she remembers this characteristic of her mother and realizes that she has married a man who goes through the same mood swings. The adult child is still holding her breath.

Subtle energetic patterns are buried deep within the neurological network of each of us. They dictate the ebb and flow of oxygen, minerals, messages, and other forms of biological energy to every cell of the body. We are born with a basic set of patterns. Over time, we imprint these basic patterns with our own idiosyncrasies. For example, in times of stress a man may unconsciously restrict the blood flow to his pancreas. The production of essential enzymes may then lag. Stress becomes a trigger for digestive problems. Chronic sluggishness and digestive stagnation develops in the digestive tract after years of responding to stress in the same way. Too many of these detrimental habit patterns are out of our awarenesses, hiding within us at the subconscious level.

Whether general lifestyle addictions (such as work patterns, recreational patterns, eating habits and drug-using patterns) or more subtle lifestyle addictions (such as deeply ingrained emotional and psychological patterns), we become increasingly controlled by our mindstyles as the years pass. Repetition of the same external and internal experiences over time erodes an automatic memory into the biological system.

Physical death offers the most certain erasure of any detrimental patterning. However, as I have suggested in the introduction to this book, there are other options. Lifestyles can be altered in a pragmatic, multilevel way. Spiritual structure can be developed in order to bring about transcendence. Deeply buried patterns can be recognized and manipulated: I call the combination of these options mindstyle surgery. I have offered a detailed plan for lifestyle surgery and steps to transcendence elsewhere in this book. Lifestyle surgery is essentially a practical effort based primarily in external reality. Steps to transcendence are more focused on the internal or spiritual reality. Both of these processes are designed to build toward minor and major transcendences of pattern addiction. At the same time, there is another level on which we must work. This is at the level of biological programming, where the mind has developed a set style or pattern of information flow.

Here what I call insight or mindstyle imagery is valuable. Images of personal energy patterns, whether entirely imagined or based on scientific information, can be built (or visualized by the imagination) in the mind's eye. These fascinating images, based upon an agreement one makes with one's mind, can represent otherwise invisible and inconceivable energetic patterns. Below is an exercise I have used to explore and work with mindstyle patterning. You may want to record your own or someone else's voice slowly reading this exercise, and then play the tape back to yourself. Be certain to pause for at least one minute where you see one star (*) and three minutes at three stars (***). However you choose to hear it, be certain to enter this exercise in a relaxed state. Locate yourself in a dimly lit, private room or a warm tub.

MINDSTYLE PATTERNING EXERCISE

Find a comfortable position for your body. With your eyes closed, put your hand over an area of your body that you feel is either not well, or is not as well as you like it to be. You may want to choose a part of your body that is hurting or one that is numb or one that seems to be less connected to you than the rest of you. If you cannot select such an area of your body, just pick any spot and put your hand on it. Hold your hand there and become aware of whatever you think of as energy in your body under your hand. Now let your hand rest there for a while...just let your mind begin to see into that part of your body. Look for energy. If you see nothing, just pretend that you see energy. [*]

If you have seen or imagined what you think of as energy — whatever this means to you — and this energy is moving, follow the path of this energy with a very slow moving fingertip. Use the hand you rested on the area of your body that you first selected. Note very carefully where this energy changes character, where it disappears, where it gets stuck.

If you feel that you are unable to find this energy, just use your imagination. Make something up. Let yourself see what you imagine you would see if you saw your energy....sparks or stars or blurry balls of light or a lion or a slug or whatever you choose to see.

Now, slowly find an area in which your energy either disappears, gets stuck or changes to an unpleasant color. Go there with your fingertip, being certain that your fingertip never leaves the surface of your body. You can press your fingertip into your flesh where the energy runs deep....

Go into this area. Using both hands now, pull the unpleasant or dead-ended energy out of your body. Feel it. Examine it. If you do not like it, pull it and everything connected to it out of your body. Use both hands to do this surgery. If you are disgusted or want to pretend that you smell a putrid smell as you do this, make a face to go with that feeling.

[*]

When you feel finished, move your finger slowly to another area of your body. It can be close to or far from the first location. Find the energy. Follow its same motion. If you do not like the energy, remove it. Do the same work in this new area of your body.

[***]

Move to another area. Do the same work again. You are house cleaning. Your body is your home. As you continue this process, begin to try to find energy that moves well and pleases you. This energy may be in or outside of your body. Again and again, replace the putrid energy with the pleasing energy you have found. You can pull energy in from outside your body any time you choose to.

[***]

When you are complete, survey your body and then open your eyes.

I have used this exercise on myself as well as with people suffering from a variety of psychological and physical afflictions. The value of such an exercise is that it calls upon our creative faculties to gain access to information about ourselves—information usually hidden from our conscious minds. The exercise, in itself, cannot be said to eliminate an actual neurological program. It can, however, assist its user in (a) becoming aware enough of the problematic programming (the energetic pattern and its chain of psychological and biological associations) to begin to work on it; (b) learning a method that, albeit may, in the beginning, have only temporary effects, provides pain and stress relief and concentration; (c) developing an intuitive method of intervening in ongoing deeply ingrained patterning that may be detrimental, of doing intuitive surgery on oneself; and (d) practicing, at the same time, a combination of creative imagery, active meditation, and deep concentration.

I find this exercise useful in exploring implicit pattern addictions behind drug (including alcohol, nicotine, and caffeine) addiction, eating addiction, depression, habitual gesturing and ticks, chronic pain, digestive problems, serious illnesses and other afflictions. With practice, users of this method can work on themselves at a very deep level. Mindstyle surgery improves in acuity with practice.

Part V

Transcending the Confines of Your Macrocosm

Give me your tired, your poor, your huddled masses
yearning to breathe free...
—Motto of the militant antismoker

13

The Family Affair

Whether it is drug addiction, overeating, or a much more subtle energy pattern addiction, the addicted individual is actually part of an addicted system. Even the most subtle, implicit pattern addictions begin developing at home, amid family life.

Because an examination of chemical dependence within families demonstrates this relationship between personal patterns and family patterns, I will spend much of this chapter using the relationship between families and drug addiction as an example. As you read through sections that discuss communication, lies, grudges, and hurts, you can substitute for drug addiction any other explicit or implicit pattern addiction. Think about the way children are programmed by their parents as they experience the same emotional scripts again and again. Family communication and energy expression patterns are woven deeply into the human biocomputer and are difficult to reprogram later on.

CHEMICAL DEPENDENCE

Chemical dependence is one of the most blatant and pervasive addictions on the planet. People of all ages get into trouble with drugs and alcohol. Children *in utero* are exposed to the highs and lows of white sugar, caffeine, nicotine, alcohol, cocaine, and other drugs when their pregnant mothers take these chemicals into their biological systems. While drugged with a stimulant such as sugar, caffeine, or cocaine, the fetus may increase its activity or become disturbed. When the stimulant is a vasoconstrictor such as caffeine, nicotine, or cocaine, the veins and arteries in the mother's body constrict and sharply reduce the flow of oxygen into the womb. When alcohol is consumed by the mother, fetal alcohol effects and defects may result.

Childhood is a time when foods with sugar and caffeine are tasted and frequently consumed in large quantities. These *psychoactive* compounds are provided by adults who either cannot say no or do not understand that children can develop sugar and caffeine dependencies. In some cases, parents actually use these dietary drugs—the psychoactive compounds found in food and beverages—to control their children. "If you are good, I'll buy you a candy bar," or "If you eat all of your dinner, you can have cake for dessert."

When parents complain that "My children just won't calm down enough to go to bed without their ice cream," they are revealing that their children have become dependent on the effects of sugar on their young bodies in order to calm down. Sugar causes a brief increase in energy, which is then followed by the calming release of seratonin in the brain, accompanied by a depressive drop in blood sugar levels.

As children grow older, they see their parents eating poorly, smoking, drinking, and using various other drugs. Then they see and hear countless advertisements showing happy and attractive people eating sugar-filled foods, smoking cigarettes, and drinking alcohol. Given that children have been born and raised in a chemical society, it is not surprising that they face the risk of becoming chemically dependent as adolescents and, later on, as adults. It is also difficult to sort out patterns of chemical use from other more implicit pattern addictions, because almost all of us have been influenced toward a high use of drugs (dietary and nondietary, legal and illegal) in our systems.

Adolescents and even adults feel social or peer pressure to "do what everyone else is doing," to "fit in" and, at an increasingly younger age in this materialistic society, to "keep up." Especially among pre-teens and teenagers, the desire not to stand out as odd or different may be a prime motivation to experiment with, and even regularly use, alcohol and other drugs. The sense of social pressure begins at a tragically early age. Unfortunately, the younger people are when they first experiment with both legal and illegal drugs, the greater the likelihood that they will have trouble with drugs later on.

Parents struggle with their children's and teenagers' desire to experiment and to respond to media and peer pressure. Yet parents often undermine their struggles by simultaneously creating the poor nutritional standards and types of dietary intake that render young people susceptible to biological cravings for drugs. After all, a childhood of high sugar consumption programs a young person's body to accept chemically induced highs and lows. To use drugs such as alcohol and cocaine to achieve highs and lows later on in life is simply to switch drugs or to add another drug to the list of those already being taken through the diet. The chemicals may be different, but the process is exactly the same.

HAVEN IN A HEARTLESS WORLD?

The ideal family has been described as a "haven in a heartless world." Yet for many of us, family life is no haven. On the contrary, it is often heartless and hypocritical. How can parents protect their children from being lured into chemical prisons, when they, the parents, are already imprisoned themselves? How many parents who smoke or drink or use other drugs attempt to tell their own children not to? How many parents criticize drug use and then unwittingly provide their children with magazines and take them to movies that glorify the use of alcohol and drugs? How many parents have time to notice the confused messages regarding drug use that they are sending their children? Given that we are faced with the chemicalization of our biosphere that I mentioned in Chapter 1, we must see that emotional and spiritual connection is needed to preserve individuals in the face of this chemical onslaught. But, many parents do not have the time to create a *heart-full* family environment instead of a heartless one. And of those parents who have the time or who make the time, how many really know how to bring about a sense of family as a haven of humanity in their homes?

Parents are confronted by the demands of adulthood: being breadwinners, home managers, child bearers, child raisers, and, at the same time, being fulfilled people. When a morning has been tiring, a coffee break may *seem* to replenish one's energy. When a day has been difficult, a drink at the end of the day may *seem* to make an hour happy.

The only answer that seems obvious is that no individual gets into trouble all by himself or herself. Whether people live with their families or not, whether they are children, teenagers or adults—their conditions are always a family affair. This means that transcendence of addiction is a family affair. The system that has locked the problem in place must release its individual members to grow, change and transcend.

THE SYMPTOMS AND EFFECTS
OF FAMILY DRUG PROBLEMS

A family feels the effect of one of its member's drug problem whether or not it officially, that is, explicitly, knows about the problem. Hidden drug problems make themselves evident via lies and communication break-downs, and in the development of grudges, hurts, and co-addictions. Even when the family knows about the problem, when the problem is not hidden, when one of its members' use is visible, these and other symptoms can still surface. Let's examine some of the behaviors characteristic of the *drug problem family*.

LIES

Lies take many forms. Some are more visible than others; these are the *obvious* lies. Others are more difficult to detect. They are *hidden*. Sometimes a person lies so often that lying becomes a way of life. These are *continuous* lies.

Obvious Lies

Obvious lies are easy to spot. If Johnny says, "I was with Mark at his house until midnight last night," when Mark was at your house with you waiting for Johnny until midnight, it is obvious Johnny is not telling the truth. But watch out! Just because this lie is obvious does not mean that it is easy to understand or respond to. Many families need a great deal of practice in the confrontation of obvious lies. Fortunately, though, although obvious lies can be extremely frustrating, they are relatively innocuous.

Hidden Lies

Hidden lies are insidious. They do their damage without revealing their presence. One of the most dangerous aspects of the hidden lie is that family members often "allow" a lie to remain hidden by choosing not to acknowledge its presence. Sometimes obvious lies are simply ignored. In other circumstances, when a family knows that something is "not quite right" but is not clear what lie is being told, the family may choose to "look the other way." Certainly some hidden lies are very deeply hidden. These lies may not come out—become obvious—until a crisis forces them to the surface. Perhaps Dad only goes on a drinking binge when he is away on his fishing trips. By the time he gets home, he has dried out and recovered from his hangover. He may not have caught any fish, but it is a standard family joke, "what a terrible fisherman Dad is." Finally, Dad has a serious boating accident as a result of his drinking. The hidden lie about his alcohol problem may then, in this time of crisis, be revealed.

Continuous Lies

In a family with a drug or alcohol problem, an array of obvious and hidden lies can easily develop into a stream of continuous lies. Over time a terrible confusion arises from the continuous lying. Lies are told to cover lies, and more lies are built over those lies. New lies cover old ones, weaving a web of deceit. It becomes very difficult to figure out what is the truth. It also becomes difficult to stop lying. Family members may reach a point where they know nothing about each other. They lose touch with each other, lose an awareness of each other's feelings, fears, and aspirations. They lose the ability to confront each other with the truth. When one or more family members gets into trouble with drugs, the entire family may become enmeshed in continuous lies. The family acts like a family of ostriches who, when threatened, put their heads into the sand so they won't have to face reality. They would rather be blinded by lies than know the uncomfortable truth.

This desire to avoid the truth is apparent in two more common types of lies: *excuses* and *denial.*

Excuses As Lies

A family with a drug problem will often find that one member of the family is constantly making excuses for himself, or for some other member of the family. These excuses help to direct the attention away from the real problem. They are lies.

Denial As Lies

Creeping denial invades the family that does not want to see the drug problem of one or more of its members. "Our children do *not* use drugs. Do you Dick and Jane?"

"Of course we don't, Mom and Dad. And neither do you." Although denial can be a very obvious hidden lie, it is often the most difficult to expose because of the implicit cooperation that every member of the family is lending to the lie.

COMMUNICATION BREAKDOWN

Every single lie, whatever type it may be, results in noncommunication. Whether caused by lies or other difficulties of expression, families with drug problems suffer from many forms of broken communication.

Lack of Communication

"Hello. No time to talk. Good-bye. I'm late, I'm late, I'm late." This is a typical scenario in far too many families. Family members rush around like mad hatters—rushing to work, rushing to school, rushing through family meals, and generally rushing away from each other. Little or no effort is made to communicate and share feelings. In many cases even simple communication, such as "I'll pick you up at four o'clock" or "Dinner is at six o'clock" or "I'll be home at eight," is never made. Lack of communication has become so very common that most people have adjusted to it and no longer find it at all unusual.

Inadequate Communication

Even when communication does occur in a drug problem family, it can be inadequate. "I told you to be home by six," say the mother. "I didn't hear you," replies her son. "That's your problem. No dinner for you now." "Who cares? I had two milkshakes while I waited for you to pick me up. You never came." "You didn't tell me you needed a ride." "Yes I did." "Next time, tell me when I'm within earshot." This kind of conversation is inadequate in that it does not express the fact that one person was wondering where the other person was and was concerned for his welfare, while that person was hurt that no one came to pick him up. Inadequate communication is when feelings and facts are buried under accusations and counteraccusations.

Confused Communication

Reality is further distorted when communication becomes confused. Family members who deal with other family members when they are craving a drink or drugs, are high on alcohol or drugs, or are experiencing hangover or withdrawal symptoms, may find their communication confused. The family member with a drug problem may change his or her mind or mood or entire personality several times a day, week, or month. The only consistency in a drug user's behavior is consistent inconsistency. This can be frightening, as users cannot be trusted to be consistent in their reactions. One minute they will be loving and kind to the members of their families, and next they can be threatening and cruel. Confused communication can lead others to become confused communicators in order to fit in. It can also plant the seeds of deep emotional disturbance in children and adolescents—seeds that may emerge later in adult life as deep neuroses.

GRUDGE DEVELOPMENT

Lies and broken communication lead to unexpressed, partially expressed, or indirectly expressed pain and anxiety. When this hurt is not fully expressed, the person who has been hurt is likely to develop a grudge.

Private Grudges

A private grudge is a strange thing, a stuffed away, unexpressed emotion that is always un-stuffing itself and breaking out in stiff, cold or angry ways. Grudges develop slowly, when communication continues to fail and lies, pain, and confusion compound. Many children grow up feeling that their siblings or their parents have grudges against them although "no one ever talked about it" and nothing was ever done that was hurtful enough to prove that a grudge actually existed.

Public Grudges

Some grudges become public in ways that are obvious. A least favored or always blamed member of the family may be the subject of a public family grudge. This person often develops private grudges in response and retaliation to family members' grudges against him or her. Using drugs without telling anyone may be one way of acting out a private grudge. On the other hand, using drugs despite the fact that "everyone knows about it and disapproves" can be a public grudge bearing act.

HURTS

Every member of a drug problem family is hurt by the family's addiction.

Obvious Hurt

Some of the hurt is visible in the forms of health problems, car accidents, domestic violence, tears at the table, and so on.

Blatant Hurt-Back

"You hurt me, I'll hurt you back." This is "an eye for an eye," tit-for-tat, type of hurt. It too is very obvious, but it can last for years and be extremely destructive.

Buried Hurt

But even more dangerous is hurt that has been buried. Adult children of alcoholics and addicts may go through half their lives before discovering and learning to express their *buried hurt*. By then, they have made buried hurt a part of their deep patterning or programming and must work very hard to transcend it. Too often buried hurt is directed against oneself before it can be expressed.

Secret Hurt-Back

Many people who have buried hurt express it through *secret hurt-back*. Private grudges, lies, and more direct but still secret acts like theft, damage, and gossip—these are all manifestations of secret hurt-back. But the most secret of hurt-backs is hidden self-destruction. Families may not notice that one of their members is on a self-destruct path until the destruction has reached a crisis stage. This is often the case with eating disorders and drug addiction.

FAMILIAL CO-ADDICTION

Over a period of time, families with drug problems begin to get used to living with lies, broken communications, grudges, and hurts. Some families even become dependent on these twisted ways of relating to each other. When this happens the family is experiencing *familial co-addiction*. This is a detrimental and implicit pattern addiction shared by all family members.

Simple Co-Addiction

No form of co-addiction is simple. I use the word *simple* to indicate, not that the relationship is easy to understand, but that the family has only one "identified patient," that is, one person whom the family admits has a problem. The characteristics of simple co-addiction include:

DEPENDENCE: While only one person may be directly dependent on drugs, other family members are dependent on the "fact" that "the addict is the one with the problem, not the rest of us."
ATTENTION: All of the family's attention is paid to the person who has the most visible problem—the addicted individual.

TIME: Family time is organized, and more often disorganized, around the addicted member's drug problem.

MONEY: Family money is consumed by the *problem*, either in buying drugs, paying for treatment or medical attention, paying for damages, or spending money as an activity to relieve the family from its stress of addiction.

CONFUSED FEELINGS: Family members who depend on the addicted member to have all the problems in the family become confused about *their own* problems and feelings.

Compound Co-Addiction

When more than one member of the family is addicted to drugs or has another unhealthy habit, the family's simple co-addiction is compounded. All of the lies, broken communications, grudges, and hurts are multiplied many times over. And each of the five characteristics of simple co-addiction that we just listed becomes even more pronounced.

PRACTICAL DIFFICULTIES AND SIMPLE CATASTROPHES

Over time, a family with a drug problem finds it more and more difficult to function. Practical difficulties compound and lead to simple catastrophes. What does this mean?

Practical Difficulties

The basic function of a family is to provide *protection* (food, clothing, and shelter), *organization* (management of time, money, and the family's living environment), *socialization* and *development* (teaching values and socially acceptable behavior, and preparing members to "learn" in school and "earn" at work) and finally *love* (however intangible that may be). Practical difficulties arising in drug problem families are (a) problems of *protection*, such as dinner not being served, inadequate nutrition, poorly dressed children, or things around the house falling into a state of disrepair; (b) problems of *organization*, such as a sense that everyone is always late, that there is never enough time for anything, that money is not budgeted or that the house is messy, chaotic, and eventually dirty; (c) problems of *socialization* and *development*, such as children being poorly mannered, developing behavioral problems, and/or falling behind in school.

Problems of Love and Practical Catastrophes

Destruction is the process by which the *structure* of something falls apart. When practical problems compound, they lead to practical catastrophes. Family life grinds to a halt. Enough practical catastrophes compounded together will *destroy* a family. In this case, love loses out to chaos.

Faltering Attention

When a parent is experiencing a drug problem, the children suffer from inconsistent and often entirely nonexistent attention to their needs, in addition to many of the practical difficulties just described. At first, addicted parents anguish over the situation, too. But if changes are not made soon, the worst can happen. As all of these difficulties begin to *break* the family down, everyone suffers from a general waning of care and love. Eventually nothing is left but little bits of what was once a real family.

Fading Heart

The drug problem family is no "haven in a heartless world." When its core is eaten away, love fades. The family's soul dies. Even going home for dinner may become a painful or painfully empty prospect. Many family members begin to function automatically, even robotically, as a means of coping with the pain and emptiness. Some family members hurt themselves or others or get physically sick as an expression of their pain. As the heart of the family begins to fade, family members die inside—little by little.

> **THE FAMILY IS A SYSTEM
> THAT REPRESENTS AND AFFECTS
> THE ENCOMPASSING SOCIAL SYSTEM
> AND, THEREFORE, AS THE FAMILY'S HEART FADES,
> THE WORLD AROUND IT BECOMES EVEN MORE HEARTLESS.
> FAMILIES WITHOUT HEART LEAD TO SOCIAL SYSTEMS WITHOUT
> HEART.**

So how do we affect societal change? Let us begin with the family. No family member is an island. The family is a system. Its whole is greater than the sum of its parts. When any one family member transcends addiction, other family members must either change or try to stay the same. Those who change break out of the rigid addictive pattern their family is ensnared in. They transcend the Catch 22 of the drug problem family; that is, "We want you well, but we also want you sick, because we *need* you to be well, but we also *need* you to be sick, because the family must change and get well to survive, but the family must stay the same— stay sick to retain its identity. Because if we change, we will never again be *us*—we will be different." Families, just like organizations, tend to want to stay the same— *to preserve the status quo*—even if change will be for the better. This is why so many families with drug problems cling to their paradoxical holding patterns. This is why when an addicted member of a family attempts to break his or her addiction, other members of the family will often do everything in their power to sabotage the efforts—just so everyone will *stay the same.*

When parents and spouses of addicted people claim that they want the addicted person to "get well," they must be ready to make the behavioral, nutritional, economic, social, and emotional changes necessary for a drug free family, and they must also be willing to see all that they have done to help create a drug problem in their family.

Drug abuse *is* a *chemical* family affair. When it comes to chemical dependence, the affair does not end at the family's boundaries. All of society is affected. And, in turn, all of society affects the family, creating the environment for the family's drug problems. The same is true for most pattern addictions, including eating, spending, emotional, sexual, and illness patterns. These are all family affairs.

This means that, just as families must release their members from rigid holding patterns, societies must release their individual members and families from the rigid societal holding patterns that resist transcendence. Can an entire society transcend? Yes. Just remember that even the largest wave is composed of millions and millions of drops of moving water. Social change is built upon the groundswell of personal change.

14

The Politics of Addiction: Information Breakdown

$\mathbf{E}$verything each one of us does is a political act. This is because every individual is an important component of a larger system. When full information fails to flow from one part of the system to its other parts, the system is in trouble. The breakdown, distortion or blockage of this vital information flow results in systematic malaise and eventually disease. This is equally true for biochemical, cellular, psychological, ecological, economic, political, and social systems. Especially in the case of drug addiction, but also in the case of all pattern addiction, individuals who are stuck in a destructive pattern are actually manifesting an information breakdown in our entire social system. Their pattern addictions are our pattern addictions. Their problems are our problems. They are stuck because they do not have adequate information regarding their predicament and possible routes of release from it.

THE POLITICS OF HEALING

The process of breaking addiction to a destructive pattern is a revolutionary experience for an individual. It also has revolutionary implications for society, because transcending addiction calls for fundamental changes in the way that an addicted person sees the world. For an addicted world to transcend addiction, the human race must see all of reality with new eyes.

When people change their world views, they inevitably affect the lives of the people around them. Through this process, every time an addiction is transcended, there are political ramifications.

So, as hundreds of thousands of citizens are treated for explicit pattern addictions such as chemical dependence and overeating, the people and organizations that treat these addicted individuals are wielding extraordinary political power—affecting the world view of their clients. They are encouraging a large number of individuals to undergo *radical* changes in their behaviors and mind-sets. When these individuals reenter society they go on to affect their friends, relatives, and co-workers. They vote for elected officials and buy consumer goods. They raise healthy children and form a large part of the future. Indeed, recovering, *discovering* addicts can become a powerful political force if they are mobilized. And if we expand the group of addicted persons to include many of those suffering from other pattern-based psychological and physical afflictions, we have a massive army of persons who can march ahead of society and lead the way down the path of transcendence.

Is their political potential at the mercy of the treatment community?

Well, yes and no. There are many, many caring and concerned members of the health care community who are actively seeking to aid their clients and patients in the struggle to transcend addictions and afflictions. But the sad truth is that much of the health care community has become mired in the "traditional" conception of the addicted and afflicted person's path and plight. As a result, the health establishment has become complacent and comfortable in its insinuations that:

- Only members of the health care establishment can diagnose a health problem.
- The diagnosis that the health care establishment makes is the only diagnosis possible and the only diagnosis that is correct.
- Observed symptoms have only certain, predetermined, official diagnoses.
- The treatment of the symptom called for by a diagnosis is the only correct treatment.
- All symptoms are exactly the symptoms they appear to be.
- If the health care establishment does not see the underlying implicit pattern addiction, it is not there.
- When what appears to be the same symptom turns up in two different individuals, both individuals are treatable in the same way.
- Alternative forms of treatment are unnecessary.
- Only those exhibiting the symptoms need treatment.
- The designated treatment will work.

- The original symptoms will be eased or will disappear when the malady is ameliorated or eliminated.
- If things get better, the prescribed *treatment* is working; if things stay the same or get worse, the *patient* is not working, i.e., not properly following the prescribed treatment.

But these claims are not true. Think about it. A lot of doctors and hospitals and insurance companies have a financial stake in maintaining old, well-established perceptions. Economic bodies like corporations buy health insurance for their employees in bulk. Insurance companies pay for traditional forms of treatment because that is the type of coverage that companies will buy; and companies buy this coverage because that is what the insurance companies will pay for. Vast profits would be lost if the diagnosis and subsequent treatment of chemical dependence or other health afflictions changed radically. By controlling the diagnostic and treatment processes, the health establishment has a stranglehold on the way we think about addiction and all illnesses. Healing has become secondary to maintaining a profit margin. Old ideas die hard, especially when loss of dollars is involved. Instead of seeking radical transformation in the definition and diagnosis of mental and physical afflictions, including chemical dependence, the health establishment perpetuates its diagnostic monopoly.

And so we continue to suffer from an information breakdown. Information regarding the true nature of pattern addictions does not circulate. It cannot circulate easily. How would the establishment adopt a revised diagnosis of pattern addiction for most illnesses?

For example, in recent decades, it has become painfully obvious that drug addiction is not the problem the health establishment has defined it as being. Diagnosis has a political component. We should be diagnosing the entire global society, not separate individuals. Until we are willing to face this global diagnosis, we are at war with truth. We are experiencing massive societal denial about chemical dependence and about all underlying pattern addiction in the same way that individual addicts experience denial when they say they are not addicted. The entire species is addicted to its implicit patterns.

FREE WILL AND THE ADDICTED SOCIETY

Let's continue our focus on chemical dependence for the moment, because it is easier to understand the ramifications of an explicit addiction than it is even to see the pervasive presence of implicit pattern addiction. Could it be that in some subtle way our global society is working to keep large numbers of its members dependent on chemicals or similarly addicted to other detrimental patterns? Are we biotechnology at its finest, or biotechnology gone wrong?

Think about the implications of your own addictions. There is a little addict person inside you. He lurks deep down in your subconscious, waiting for an opportunity to "drive" you—to commandeer your decision making processes. You may think that you live free, but you are deluding yourself. You are actually a prisoner of your little addict person, and he will eventually find and exploit your weakness—if he hasn't done so already. How readily we succumb to the subtle but continuous diminishing of human freedom when we trade away personal freedom for pattern addiction.

To relinquish the freedom of responsibility, of self-control, to an automatic addiction is, in fact, a cop-out. Rather than cope with reality, you let your little addict person feed you mechanisms that muffle your consciousness, stifle the stresses of life along with your alertness, offer you illusions of relief—vacations from attention demands.

Eventually, the wonderful and usually subconscious lie of pattern addiction turns sour—but by then it is too late. You have become a slave to your addiction. Only an internal revolution of phenomenal proportions can set you free again. Transcendence is this revolution.

Understanding what it means to say "I am an addict" is a difficult process. Feeling what it takes to know "I am an addict" is painful. Acknowledging that you are an addicted individual precipitates a sense of *ought to*—a pressure to break the cycle of pattern addiction. That *ought to* begins to lurk in the innermost recesses of the self, where the free will and the living soul have retreated.

The anguish of exorcising an invader, of ripping out an automatic pattern that has taken you over, that you have embedded within your own nervous system, makes it easier to stay with the addiction than to cut it out of your life. Breaking the unwieldy, intractable habit cycle seems as impossible as turning the tide or halting an avalanche. The myopic and eventually blind security of pattern addiction seems relatively comfortable when you are staring into the face of harsh reality—personal responsibility and freedom. For the pattern-addicted individual there is always the fear that reality will hurt more than addiction. Mindless obedience often appears more comfortable than profound change, and slavery safer than freedom.

Surrender to any damaging pattern addiction is a countersoul experience. Addiction enables an individual to undergo soul death—a false and yet tragic death—an unwillingness to let detrimental programming die. Progressive addictive behavior is a process of surrender in which *free will is eroded* until the will of the individual eventually disappears. A healthy death of the sort described in the introduction to this book becomes nearly impossible. Independent decision-making capabilities are commandeered by robotic, mechanical tendencies. The human bio-technology rolls over and plays machine. Soul dead.

As free will and self-control die, *a vacuum of vulnerability* is left inside the mind of the addicted individual. This vacuum sucks in outside agents; chemicals, other people. Opportunistic physical diseases, social forces and organizations move in and take control. They take over the decision-making processes that were once controlled by the free will of the individual. When this happens, we surrender our basic human rights to *individual power*, to the realization of our own spirituality, and therefore to our collective humanity.

The sad truth about the advance of pattern addiction is that it has prepared us to be controlled—not only to relinquish our free will, but worse, *to forget what free will is*. This is the most insidious politic of addiction. We are denying our own freedom when we fail to acknowledge the larger picture. Blind denial is a losing stance. *It is time to become conscious and to pay attention.* It is time to actively ferret out our most damaging implicit as well as explicit pattern addictions. It is time to transcend.

EPILOGUE
Lifehealing:
Freeing the Dying Heart

Highly sensitive, feeling people are an endangered species. Their hearts are hiding, dying. Their lives are wounded. They are being forced into chemicalization and mechanization. They retreat from a high degree of sensitivity (sensitivity to the stress, hassle, and pain of modern life) to save themselves. But then, they risk killing off their souls. Without contact, without inspiration, life can be very difficult. Some of us break down. Some of us get sick. Some of us die. And some just live the limbo of soul death, the most false and unhealthy death of all.

The pattern-addicted individual has made little and big decisions, over a period of time, to trade away the freedom of self-control in order to avoid and to numb the pain of living. In so doing, addicted people have selected the path without heart. They have decided to live like machines—or practically like machines. They have become creatures of habit—increasingly mechanical men. The life within their souls is draining away. And a rock feels no pain. Nor does a machine.

Ultimately, it is love that can free the addicted person and turn humanity away from the path of the robot. Seek the highest path for your own heart. Love can transcend the intense lure of the land of no feeling—the seemingly safe but very empty place of the dead heart.

Something strange is happening to love. It is slipping away from us—all of us. Deciding to find love and to feel love again is the first step in freeing humanity's dying heart, in lifehealing. In this effort, we must all become like children taking our first steps, learning to explore the precious and fragile land of our truest feelings. In so doing, we preserve what is most human about us in an environment that pressures us to be more distant from our hearts, more machinelike, more automatic, every day. You can help us transcend. You can transcend. Transcendence is lifehealing.

Transcending Addiction
(Second Edition)
APPENDIX ONE

Survival and Counter-Survival

We are all about survival. Or are we? Survival is why we live. Or is it? We have to wonder. Although our personal experiences in our daily lives may not tell us this directly, survival of the species appears to be what most of our behavior is about. After all, we sense, on some deep level, that without the survival of the species, we as individuals have no future and will cease to exist. Yet, the human brain, and the behaviors it conducts, do not always work toward survival. Sure, the human brain does its best. Yet, this human brain of ours is not coping as well as, nor evolving as rapidly as, we may need it to.

At the center of this quagmire is the matter of the environment which is changing at an ever faster pace than is the brain which directs us as we live in the environment. This conflict in the rate of change between the environment and the brain may be resulting in a diminishing of the brain's ability to read essential feedback coming from the environment to the brain. The brain therefore cannot rely entirely on the modern environment to set limits. As a result, behaviors directed by the brain frequently slip into runaway mode.

The older environment regulated these behaviors (via danger, fear, pain, and hunger for example) and thereby placed greater limits on runaway behaviors driven by the brain. However, the modern environment, especially in the so-called "developed" world, offers far less in the way of these very external controls the brain evolved itself to respond to. Certainly, we do not want the dangerous external limits found in nature to resurface everywhere en mass. Yet, we need to be able to recognize signs we may be harming ourselves, perhaps even threatening our survival. How then do we proceed?

SURVIVAL?

We have arrived in these times, apparently far less able to regulate our behaviors just when we need to be far more able to regulate our behaviors. Here we are, in the modern world, in the face of opportunities for endless excess—excess in consumption of refined sugar, low quality carbohydrates, alcohol, drugs, gambling, spending, and a host of other compelling substances and activities. We feel the pull of excess, we are even drawn to it. We are confused by yet recognize this sensation. We want to turn away but too often cannot. We feel this tug of war on some very deep level. Too often we find that neither our environments nor our brains can stop us from slipping into detrimental patterns of excess and of addiction to *detrimental excess.*

Excess, runaway excess, is a mounting and potentially devastating problem loaded with the tragic flaws of hypocrisy and the failing of the human brain to set limits. Most excess has lost its purpose in modern times and in the modernized world. It seems that necessary excess now appears less and less, not even in new and valid versions of survival-oriented forms (similar to the old layer of excess fat found on an animal storing up for winter hibernation --- likely once necessary for us).

Modern people almost entirely miss the point, the survival value, of excess, yet consume to the level of excess whenever possible. While populations in some areas of the planet cannot get enough food, water, medicine, and shelter to grow and live, large portions of so-called "modernized" populations are driven to seek, to constantly seek, immediate gratification for other than survival purposes. In fact, in modern times, drives for immediate gratification that may have no actual survival value have become almost normal, for varying reasons. Not surprisingly, a great deal of modern marketing aims to stimulate these drives.

GRATIFICATION?

The drive for immediate gratification is a two-edged sword, one side true survival based need, the other side some other drive masking itself as survival based. Indeed, in the all out no-holds-barred drive for immediate gratification are found both: (a) the seeking of relief from suffering, and (b) the seeking of relief from longing for gratification.

A note here. Those who have suffered from severe migraines know what it feels like to have that intense pain finally recede—it feels good! Relief from suffering is surely a form of pleasure, perhaps the greatest pleasure there is. So we have one of the greatest and saddest ironies of human want. What is legitimate survival oriented **need**, and what is troubled gratification-seeking addiction? When are we confused regarding the difference? Much of the time.

This problem of the drive for desire gratification (and the distortions of this drive) is an equal opportunity, a malady affecting people of all ages, in all walks of life, in all levels of "well" being, everywhere. Hence, this monster we call problem addiction rears its ugly head everywhere we look. And it reaches to great and seemingly unlikely extremes, for example to street children in various parts of the world who use coca (as per cocaine) paste or sniff glue to relieve their hunger pains or ward off the cold, and to masses of children around the world, in all walks of life, exposed to drugs and alcohol prior to birth and during childhood.

Here we must force ourselves to witness (even when we may choose to deny) this reality, the modern problem addictions seizing the human population worldwide. The objects of these addictions move to the forefront—these are substances and activities many of which powerfully stimulate the pleasure and reward (reinforcement) centers of the brain to generate direct pleasure as well as the pleasure of relief from displeasure, discomfort, and suffering. The objects of these addictions can now regulate human behavior more powerfully than can the environment the brain needs to have helping it control itself. Behavioral inadequacies, inconsistencies and distortions result.

We know this, we are sensing this disturbing development. And we also know that in nature, immediate gratification is rare. Instead, nature takes its time. A primary exception to this taking of time in nature is the instance of immediate response to danger when the "fight or flight" syndrome kicks in. Fortunately, some of this mechanism remains functional in our brains today. When instinct kicks in, we instinctively respond to danger by either taking flight or fighting back. Unfortunately, many drugs and activities to which we can become addicted stimulate parts of the brain involved in this fight or flight reflex.

Furthermore, the fight or flight reflex is confused now. When the modern brain senses an actual shortage of something, or even the threat of a pause in the flow of needed resources and security, it responds to the perceived as well as actual famine (of supplies and resources, of opportunity, of power, of safety) by consuming, even consuming dangerously at times, and or expressing addictively whatever it can—no matter how counter-survival this expression may be.

Transcending Addiction
(Second Edition)
APPENDIX TWO

Need, Desire, Pleasure, Stimulation, and Risk

We indeed have planted deep within us the coding to function as creatures of habits—of habit patterns—to inherit habits via our genes and via modeling from our parents and families and cultures, and also to develop habit patterns on our own while living our lives. As if this coding function was purposefully implanted within us, in our genes (to ensure our ability to live and learn, to ensure that we function as life forms), we are built to utilize this coding function every moment of our lives. It is this function which makes it possible for us to perceive (and even define for ourselves) a reality as a given, to tell ourselves we know where we are in time and space. It is this coding function that makes it possible for us to define our reality in every way in order to live "within" it—in order to live. And yes, part of living within a given reality successfully is buying into that reality entirely, or almost entirely.

SURVIVAL RELIES ON THIS PROGRAMMING

Although quite subtle, the tendency is to form an addiction to reality itself, (or to what is perceived as reality itself), to survive. In fact, organisms such as ourselves develop beneficial adaptations to the environment—to reality—that increase the likelihood of our survival.

(We also change the environment where we can, sometimes increasing the likelihood of our survival, sometimes increasing the likelihood of our present-time survival but unfortunately failing to do the same for the long run. What a gamble changing our environment in the now, with little regard for long term consequences, is!)

We have been doing this adaptation to the environment throughout our evolution. And we have been passing on the adaptations to our environments we have developed via our genes (as well as via our cultures and traditions).

So while the brain's reward system reinforces important behaviors today, in the now—eating, drinking, sleeping, mating—this survival oriented functioning itself has been passed on to us through time and we pass this on to future generations. However—and this is a big however here—all this is predicated on the successful passing on of an adherence to a reality in which these functions work and continue to be survival-oriented. While this is a rather lofty concept, it can be brought right down to Earth with the simple example of hunting prey for dinner. In the modern so-called "developed" world, we rarely have to directly hunt and kill prey for dinner. In fact, were we to engage in this activity in our neighborhoods and cities today, we might find ourselves mistakenly applying this drive to household pets and zoo animals. Health concerns, anger and havoc could emerge.

Fortunately, we have adapted this drive to hunt and kill our prey for dinner to our modern environment and now control and even suppress this drive where necessary. By contrast, we have other drives which we need to continue today, such as the drives to sleep and to mate. Fortunately we still mate, although population and corresponding scientific pressures may be changing mating and related sexual behaviors.

Let's take the behavior of sleep as a yet more general example. We need to sleep. Fortunately we are coded to need sleep, to feel the need for sleep, and to sleep when tired. Where there may be a point in the development of the species where sleep is not required, this new adaptation will require internal genetic coding (and or external medical interventions) to ensure that whatever metabolic and behavioral changes are needed are made.

RISK AND STIMULATION AS TRIGGERS FOR GAMBLING
AND GAMBLING WITH LIFE

Focusing in on risk itself, note that various readings of and responses to the sensation of risk have evolved over time and are in play in many problem addictions today. Gambling addiction provides a case in point. Brain scans have shown that when particular men are shown erotic pictures, they are more likely to make larger financial gambles than they are when they are shown frightening or disturbing pictures (such as pictures of dangerous animals attacking). When these same men are shown something more neutral such as pictures of office equipment, they make gambles in the midrange. Brain scans reveal that when photos of snakes and spiders are shown to the men, the portion of the brain associated with pain, fear, and anger light up. Upon being shown these disturbing, even frightening pictures, the men are likely to keep their bets low, as the pain, fear and anger experienced causes the risk taking drive to minimize itself. By contrast, viewing erotic pictures results in other areas of the brain being lit up, and greater risk taking behavior (in gambling) follows. We are such vulnerable and programmable creatures.

There are numerous basic patterns we are coded to exhibit in both positive and negative ways. As is true for patterns of risk taking, many behaviors, deep virtually subconscious at their most active levels, are of value to us as we survive as a species. Yet the very coding which guides us as we live can drive us into, and hold us imprisoned in, a vicious cycle of a serious problem addiction.

In essence, most of our behaviors relate to risk, risk perception, risk assessment, risk response, risk control, risk denial, and or risk distortion. We take risks for both survival and counter survival reasons, but we do take risks. Risk taking is gambling, risking the outcome of action in the now regardless of the potential later cost of that action taken now. To make this gamble, we must either not know, or not want to know, the potential high cost of that action's outcome. Or we may know and deny what we know in order to whole-heartedly take this risk. Denial rears its ugly head. Denial of entire aspects of realities, of entire realities, looms.

REWARD RISK?

Let's return to the matter of the brain's reward system. Rewards are the positive reinforcements that, among other things, initiate and perpetuate our specific addictions, and our addictions to whole encompassing realities. Reward balances itself against risk to modulate, regulate, and ultimately to even define our behaviors, our behaviors within our realities, even our realities themselves. We are constantly weighing reward versus risk, seeking a "safe" place between these.

Transcending Addiction
(Second Edition)
APPENDIX THREE

Calling for Complete Overhaul

We humans are such sensitive, feeling organisms, so sensitive we run from the very pain we are able to feel, we seek relief from the very discomfort we are programmed to experience. Patterns of problem addictions offer us a seemingly "safe" refuge from discomfort, the illusion of a hiding place.

We can run, but we cannot hide. Pattern addiction is wired right into us. We are creatures of habit, slaves to our programming. We are chained to the very coding that makes it possible for us to survive while it also makes it possible for us to exterminate ourselves. How do we break free of this trap, this double bind, this paradox? What would a complete overhaul of our situation look like?

Most afflictions, (including but not limited to troubled addictions), are either the product of, or carry with them, problematic or troubled energy flow patterns. A rebalancing or correction in the establishing and perpetuating of patterns of neurological and other biological energy throughout the body can reduce and even alleviate many health problems. When this rebalancing is brought about, a harmful energetic pattern, the implicit and rigid pattern of the affliction, is broken, or at least made malleable, and can be rewired.

However, concerted effort must be made to effectively eliminate the negative impact of the deeper aspects of this pattern. The harmful pattern must be extinguished or at least profoundly rewritten. Without correcting the underlying and the most implicit pattern addictions, without over-riding, overcoming, and then addressing full on the power of the programming behind the troubled surface psychological behaviors and addictions, the same or similar symptoms can continue, recur, and expand. The deeper problematic pattern behind the surface problem pattern must go or be rewired.

However, surgery will not erase this deeper underlying patterning, nor will pills nor general medical interventions. This inability to permanently eliminate deep patterns is, of course, largely due to the inability of current medical and psychological technology to see the complexity and massive number of layers of patterning driving a large part of all behavior and disease.

Yet, each of us carries internally the gift of ending patterns from the inside: a kind of internal shedding must take place. The knowledge allowing us to do this is already within us. We must travel through the surface patterns down to the implicit patterns, and then down to the source patterns driving them. We know how to will ourselves to undergo a thorough transformation—A COMPLETE OVERHAUL—we just need to be reminded how. All we need to be able to do is to travel (or at least reach deep enough) into the place where we can let underlying patterning fade or die out.

SUBSTANCE ADDICTION AS AN EXAMPLE

Let's travel back up from deep deep source patterning, up through implicit patterning, all the way to the surface, the explicit patterning and addiction which we can see. Drug and alcohol or substance addiction offers one of the most tangible examples of explicit patterning. Persons addicted to substances move from: (a) "triggers," which bring out in them reflexes, urges and even "cravings"; to (b) repeat again and again the behaviors of the addiction patterning; which (c) bring out in them the use yet again of the drug or behavior to which they are addicted.

Until the pattern of this addiction is broken, the person trapped in it remains just this—trapped. A new response will interfere with the patterning, providing at least an insight into an alternative to this pattern, however it will take substantial work to hold that insight and break this deeply burned in pattern. Breaking this pattern would allow the new response to be the new way of life. This matter is central as we look to our individual and species futures. Can we learn to detect and to shed problem programming on a wide scale? Yes we can. Shedding or overcoming problem programming is central in transcendence.

THE CHOICEPOINT

Let us consider some overarching issues here:

> **Addiction to a reality**
> **defines, supports and perpetuates**
> **the reality in which**
> **the addiction to that reality exists.**

We are at a critical choice point in human evolution. We squirm with discomfort, in faint recognition of this landmark, and then we look away, denial being so soothing. Population, urbanization, institutionalization, mechanization, globalization, and other modern pressures are bringing about a profound change in the life of the individual. Depersonalization and dehumanization are encroaching upon us. Even if she or he does not see it or believe it, the individual human is receding in the face of the technological collective.

More than ever before, we are members of a large species which swarms the globe. We are witting and unwitting soldiers, drones in the army of change. We are the new working-class heroes. We each do our part to help build the mirage of progress, to manifest what we believe is the human destiny. We participate, we cooperate, because this gives our lives meaning. We are good at taking orders, especially implicit orders which are difficult to detect and question.

As we become increasingly committed to our individual roles in the development of an increasingly global social/economic order, we must be certain to remain highly conscious, to recognize the subtle trade-offs that we are making. Many of the desired outcomes of modernization are beneficial; however, we must ask ourselves if we are willing to pay their price.

This is about staying aware. Whether we are talking about addiction to a specific drug, or to a specific behavior, or to an overarching reality, **we are talking about being programmed**. We are talking about subordinating our *true selves* to what may appear to be our selves, but not be our actual selves: our programming. So do pay attention.

ARE YOU YOUR SELF OR ARE YOU YOUR PROGRAMMING?

ARE YOU YOUR SELF OR ARE YOU YOUR ADDICTIONS?

It is important to pay attention at all times, to shake off our daze, and to never to look away. In this way we will be able to override the specific evolutionary developments which make it increasingly difficult to pay and want to pay attention. Consider some of the undesirable futures depicted by science fiction writers. How close have we already come to these fictionally depicted means of mind and social control? In Yevgeny Ivanovich Zamyatin's novel, *We*, workers live in glass houses, have numbers rather than names, wear identical uniforms, eat chemical foods, and have their sex rationed by the government. The "single state" depicted in the anti-Utopian *We* uses an operation resembling a lobotomy on workers to control them.

In our culture, we are not subjected as a matter of social policy to surgical lobotomies; however, we do use drugs, television, and our denial mechanisms to lie to and "control" ourselves and our feelings. In George Orwell's novel, *1984*, torture and brainwashing are relied upon to keep the masses in line. In the nonfictional times of today, the present day, we don't need to use torture on ourselves when we are so adept at cultural brainwashing. Aldous Huxley's novel, *Brave New World* depends upon artificial biological selection and drugs to control the masses. In our real life brave new world, we are virtually able to perform conception in a jar, and genetic engineering is upon us.

But, the most shocking is that our government does not need to drug us. We willingly do this ourselves. Social control is most expedient when the subjects participate voluntarily and, better yet, when they do so unbeknownst to themselves. Does this sound a little like addiction? Yes, it does. And, it is.

The atrocities of *Brave New World* are not restricted entirely to fiction. As noted earlier, it was only centuries ago, in the early 1500s, that Spanish conquistadores conquered the Incan empire of what is now called South America. In doing so, they assumed control over the Incas' coca leaves. They changed the use of the coca leaf, which is the source of the modern drug cocaine, from a cherished right to a form of social control. The Spaniards gave coca quite liberally to the indigenous people in order to enslave them both in South America, and back in Spain where they were also taken as slaves. Under the influence of coca, the "Indios" (as they were called) were able to work harder, longer, with less food, and with less awareness of their misery. Similar to what happens in fictional accounts of futuristic controlled societies, in this culture of the past, tucked away neatly in history, the "Indios" were drugged by their "employers" or "owners" to work, to work hard, and then they were worked to death.

Are we controlled today? I would say yes, although the mechanisms are quite subtle. Take people management—crowd control—for example. The administration of drugs is less expensive and seemingly less immoral than the use of chains, whips, strait jackets. If the people who are being controlled will willingly drug themselves or engage in some activity that dazes their minds, it will not even be necessary to hire the staff to administer the drugs. When we stretch the definition of drugs (as this book has done) just a bit to include drug-like activities such as gambling, shopping, and that all favorite past time, television, we see how common outside controls are— even the voluntarily ingested audiovisual tranquilizer—television.

Although we were once outraged by the fictional *Brave New World* concept of compulsory mass psychoactive medication in a controlled society, we calmly acquiesce to massive self-medication in our free society. We do not merely acquiesce; we insist upon trying to convince ourselves that the "addiction problem" is small—that it affects only a small portion of the population—and that we are not part of it. We tell ourselves that some addictive drugs and some addictive activities are acceptable while others are not.

If we are this unclear and this dishonest about alcohol, painkillers, tranquilizers, maybe caffeine, then we are bound to be in a deep state of denial about supposed nondrugs which drug us such as television, computers, work, gambling, shopping, and the biggest and most paradoxical drug of all, the need for and drive to have money itself. We are living in such a daze, such a largely benevolent stupor, that we do not recognize how drugged, how dulled, our minds and our senses are. We do not realize how numb and drone-like, even mechanical, we are becoming. We may not realize this, we may not see ourselves making this adaptation, but we feel this deeply. We are macro-level problem addicted.

OVERHAUL IS KEY TO HEALING PATTERN AFFLICTION

Breaking troubled pattern addictions can heal a variety of maladies, most likely even diseases. After all, sickness is a problem pattern. These are all pattern afflictions. Hitting bottom, crashing into a sort of psychological death, can be utilized in healing afflictions. We need to realize this, to get it. When addicted or ill individuals arrive at any treatment or medical service, program, or facility, they should find themselves at the door to their own self-initiated mental, physical, and spiritual overhaul. To walk themselves through such a doorway—a doorway into true overhaul—to really do this, is to die a death or, better stated, is to have the problem pattern die a death.

This problem pattern death is actually a rebirth or survival of the SELF, a movement into greater free will and freedom: free of detrimental patterns which can make us problem addicted and can make us sick, past the death of these patterns. Here is the threshold of transcendence. Here is the opportunity to harvest the death of the negative patterning for the very energy needed to be free from it!

All too often, addicted and otherwise afflicted individuals find themselves standing at a door to anything but health and freedom. Most mental and physical health care services manifest a range of attitudes toward affliction, but they rarely say, "Welcome. We are fortunate to have you among us, because you are about to lead us in an exploration of the deepest level of self—mind, body and spirit. You are about to meet the challenge of addiction to hidden patterning, to understand the death of one's patterning, and in that understanding help to explore the frontiers of healing, of freedom, of human potential, of healing potential, and of the human soul. We are truly fortunate to have you among us."

Instead, addicted and even physically ill people are subtly labeled, implicitly stigmatized, treated like "sick people." They are separated from what we call "the rest of us." It is not so much a lack of expertise that is the problem with most mental and physical health care, it is a lack of understanding of what so-called "sick" individuals are all about and a lack of respect for the critical role that they play in the evolution of human health and consciousness. Like canaries going ahead of miners in a cave, testing the air for breathe-ability, reading the signs of danger, people who fall into problem addictions and other pattern sicknesses give us signs. And people who heal their problem addictions and pattern sicknesses indicate there is a way to survive the cave, to forge a new path out of the cave to a new place. The path is rewiring the SELF. The path these people reveal to us is the path of the SELF to the TRUE SELF.

Welcome to the next step in our evolution. Witness our growing abilities to consciously rewire, rewrite, our (and our species') behaviors and programmings. We do have within us the ability and will to transcend problem programming, to transcend addiction and other afflictions. We do have this ability, as individuals, and as a species. Hope is power.

Transcending Addiction
(Second Edition)
APPENDIX FOUR

Illustrations

places:	times:	feelings:	drugs:	people:
Bathrooms	Birthdays	Depression	Sugar	John
Car	Weekends	Boredom	Caffeine	Cathy
Parties	Having to do things I don't want to do	Need for excitement	Nicotine	My Kids
Motels	After work	Sexual desires	Alcohol	Anne
BARS	Before work	MAD	Marijuana	Mark
Doctor's Office	Before sex	HAPPY	Valium & Pain Pills	Dad

identified problem:

TOO MUCH ALCOHOL AND TOO MANY PILLS

and then worse feelings:

Extremely Depressed	Guilty	Nervous

Scared	Paranoid

SUICIDAL FEELING

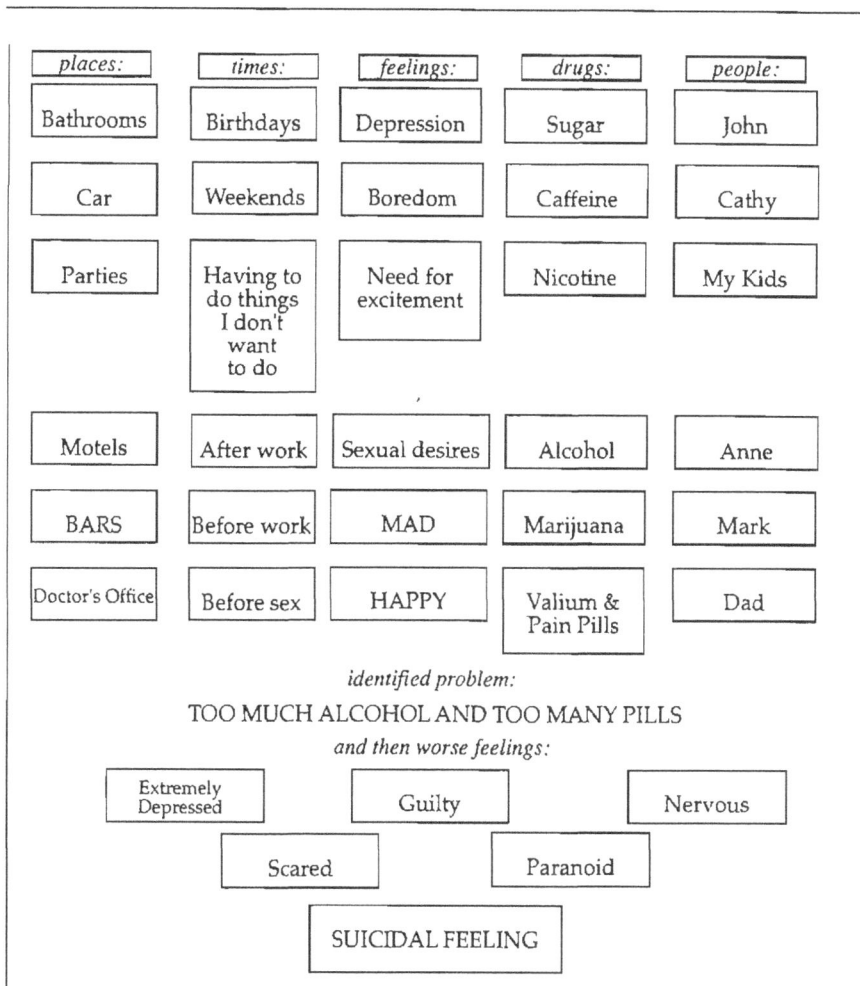

POLY-ADDICTED PERSON'S TRIGGER CHART
(Illustration courtesy of Angela Browne-Miller.)

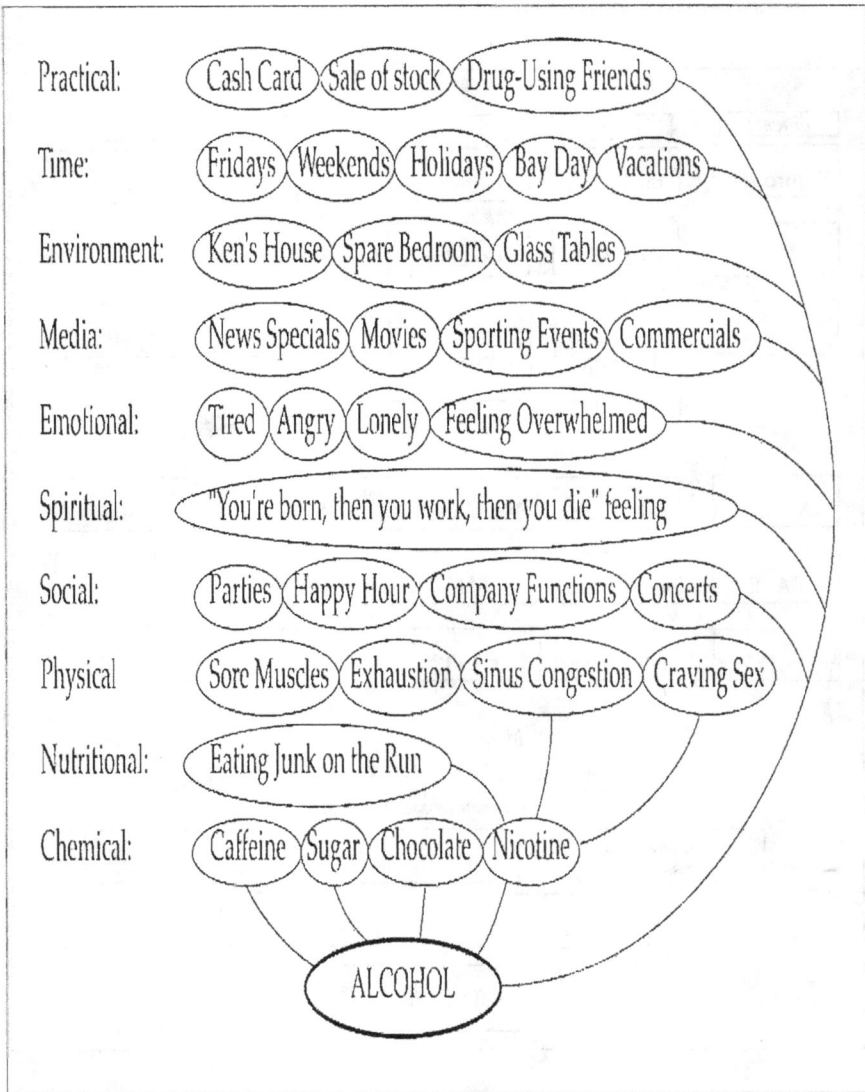

Practical: Cash Card · Sale of stock · Drug-Using Friends

Time: Fridays · Weekends · Holidays · Bay Day · Vacations

Environment: Ken's House · Spare Bedroom · Glass Tables

Media: News Specials · Movies · Sporting Events · Commercials

Emotional: Tired · Angry · Lonely · Feeling Overwhelmed

Spiritual: "You're born, then you work, then you die" feeling

Social: Parties · Happy Hour · Company Functions · Concerts

Physical: Sore Muscles · Exhaustion · Sinus Congestion · Craving Sex

Nutritional: Eating Junk on the Run

Chemical: Caffeine · Sugar · Chocolate · Nicotine

ALCOHOL

ALCOHOL USE, ABUSE, ADDICTION TRIGGER CHART
(Illustration courtesy of Angela Browne-Miller.)

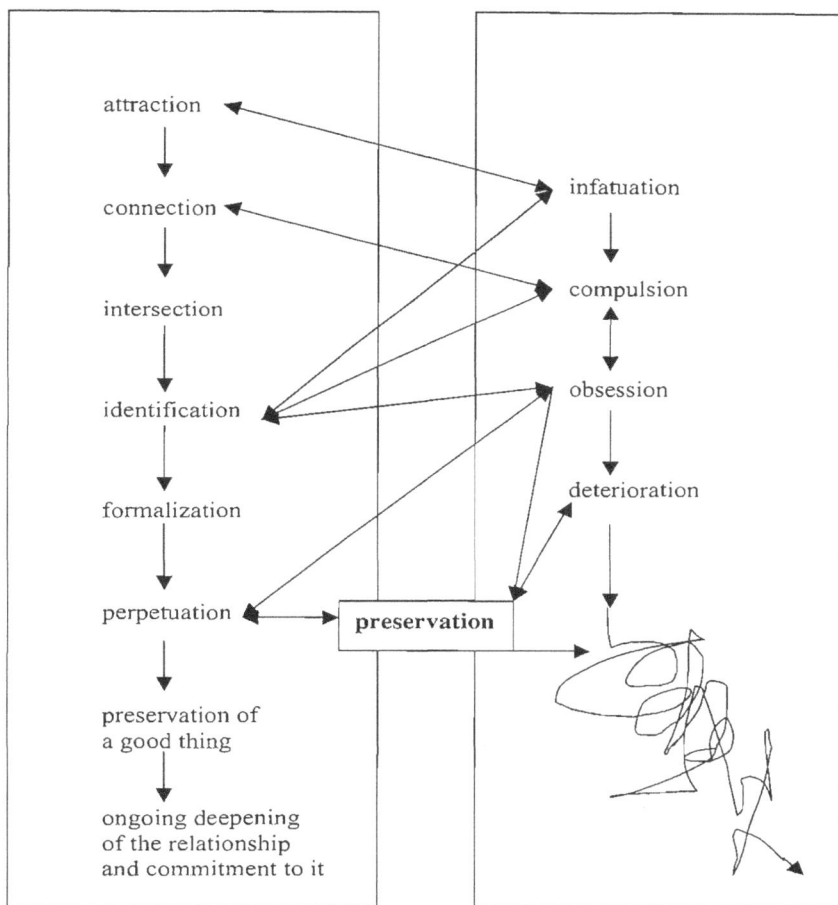

positive progression ←←←   →→→ problem progression

FROM POSITIVE TO
PROBLEM RELATIONSHIP ADDICTION PATTERN
(Illustration by and courtesy of Angela Browne-Miller.)

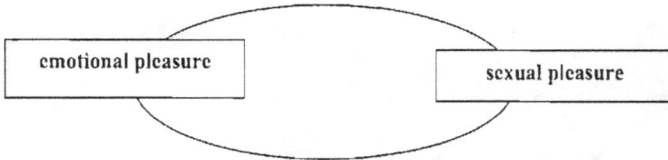

EMOTIONAL AND SEXUAL PLEASURE CYCLE

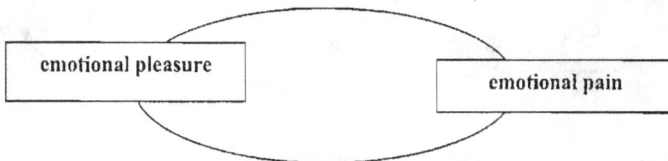

EMOTIONAL PLEASURE AND EMOTIONAL PAIN CYCLE

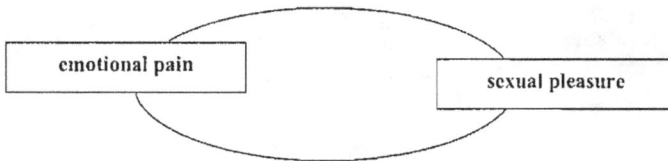

EMOTIONAL PAIN WITH SEXUAL PLEASURE CYCLE

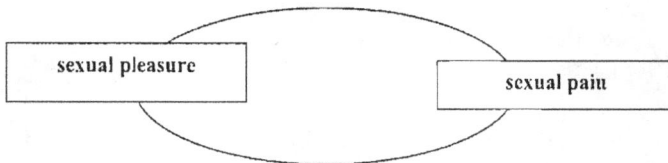

SEXUAL PLEASURE WITH SEXUAL PAIN CYCLE

PROBLEM RELATIONSHIP BEHAVIOR PATTERNS
(examples of)
(Illustration by and courtesy of Angela Browne-Miller.)

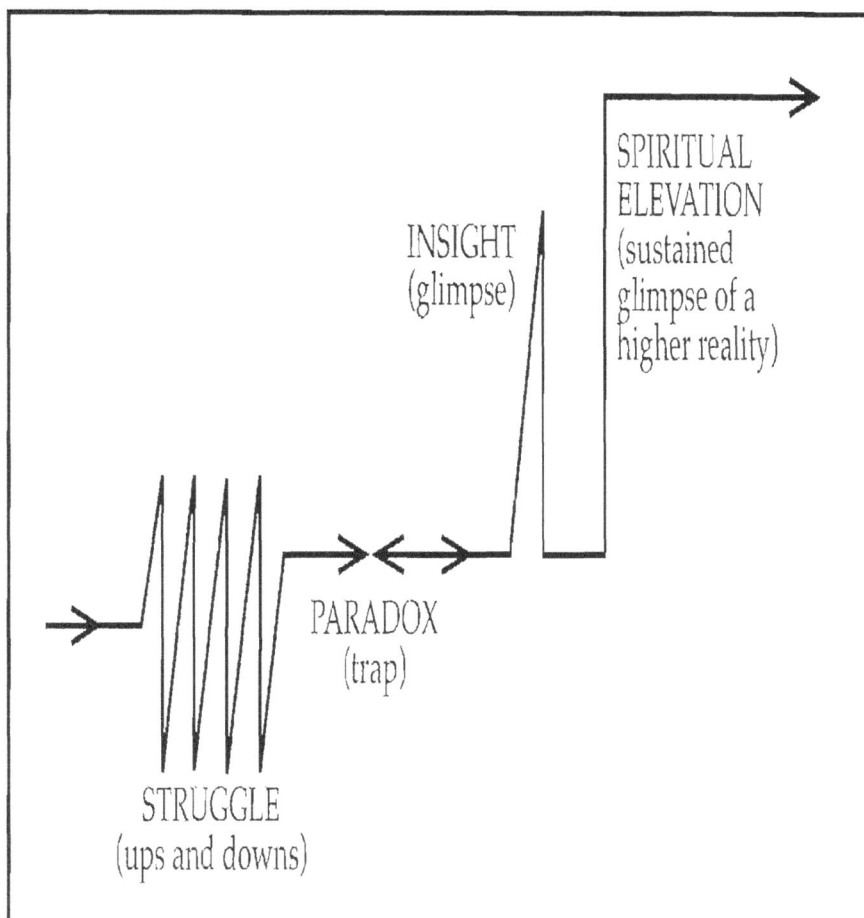

PHASES OF TRANSCENDENCE
(lliusration by and courtesy of Angela Browne-Miller.)

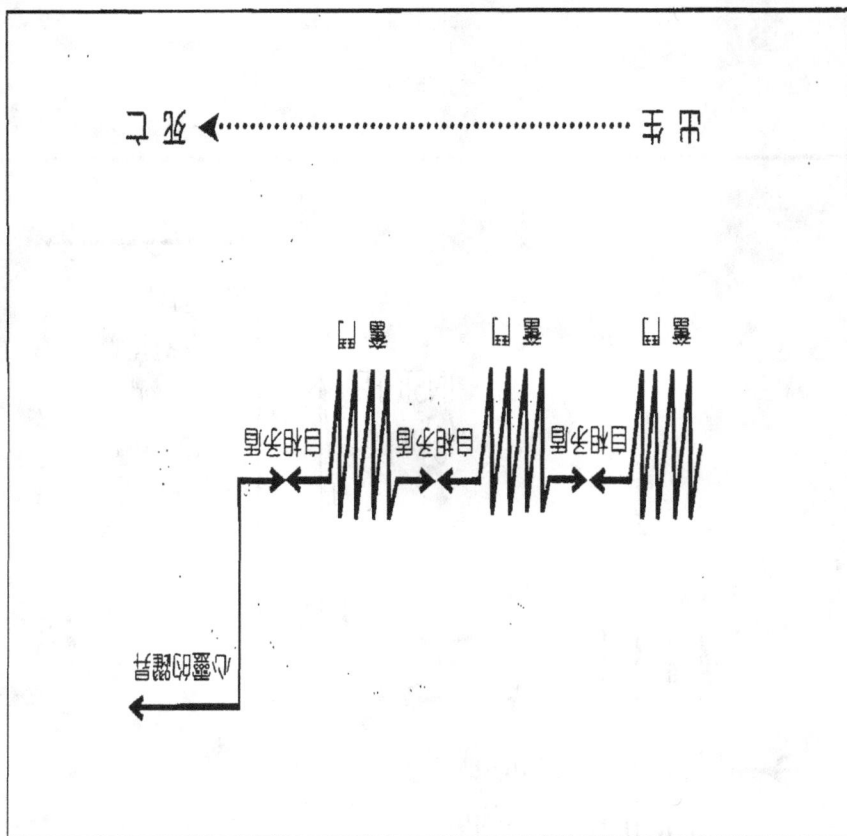

**PHASES OF TRANSCENDENCE BY ANGELA BROWNE-MILLER
PUBLISHED IN CHINA**
(Illustration courtesy of Angela Browne-Miller.)

185

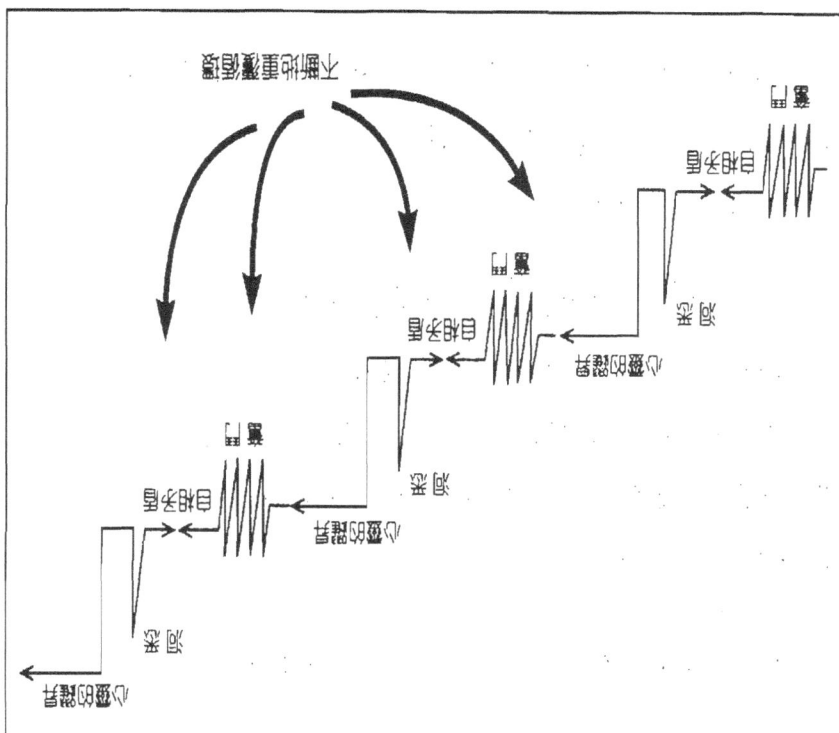

**LIFELONG
REPEATING OF THE PHASES OF TRANSCENDENCE
BY ANGELA BROWNE-MILLER
PUBLISHED IN CHINA**
(Illustration courtesy of Angela Browne-Miller.)

ABOUT THE AUTHOR

Dr. Angela Browne-Miller, also known as Dr. Angela®, founder and director of ADDICTION STOPPERS® Intensive and Follow-On Outpatient Programs, is author some forty books including: *Transcending Addiction and Other Afflictions: Life Healing* (first and second editions); *Rewiring Your Self To Break Addictions and Habits: Overcoming Problem Patterns*; and, *To Have and To Hurt: Seeing, Changing or Escaping Patterns of Abuse in Relationships*. Dr. Browne-Miller is the Set Editor of the *Praeger International Collection on Addictions*; Set Editor of the *Violence and Abuse in Society* collection; also Director of the Metaxis Institute for Personal, Social, and Systems Change, based in northern California; Director of Browne and Associates Violence, Substance Abuse, and Trauma Treatment and Prevention Program, also in northern California. Dr. Browne-Miller has been a keynote speaker at conferences around the world on addiction, violence, trauma, behavior change, and consciousness. Dr. Browne-Miller earned two doctorates and two master's degrees at the University of California, Berkeley, where she lectured in three departments for fourteen years. She has served as a U.S. National Institute of Mental Health Postdoctoral Fellow, a U.S. Department of Public Health Fellow; public relations director for Californians for Drug Free Youth; Research Education and Treatment Director for the Cokenders Alcohol and Drug Program; advisor to addiction treatment programs in the United States and several other countries; and project director on several California Department of Health abuse and violence prevention projects. She has worked in clinical and educational settings with several thousand persons addicted to, or working with persons addicted to, drugs, alcohol, sex, love, relationships, violent activities, gambling and gaming, food, and to other objects, substances and activities, and is an expert in the human mind and consciousness, and also in the psychobiological and psychosocial aspects of health, co-occurring disorders, and dual diagnoses. Dr. Browne-Miller also lectures at Alliant International University and California School for Professional Psychology in San Francisco, California. She can be reached at DrAngela@DrAngela.com

Books by the Author
Angela Browne-Miller
Also uses pen name: <u>DR. ANGELA DEANGELIS</u>

<u>Endings are Beginnings:</u>
<u>Navigating Your Hard Times Into Higher States</u>
Written by Angela DeAngelis.

<u>Embracing Eternity:</u>
<u>The Life Force Does Not Die</u>
Written by Angela DeAngelis.

<u>Healing Earth in All Her Dimensions:</u>
<u>Personal, Species and Planetary Healing</u>
Written by Angela DeAngelis.

<u>Rewiring Your Self to Break Addictions and Habits:</u>
<u>Overcoming Problem Patterns</u>
Written by Angela Browne-Miller.

<u>To Have and To Hurt:</u>
<u>Seeing, Changing or Escaping Patterns of Abuse in Relationships</u>
Written by Angela Browne-Miller.
Foreword by Arun Ghandi.

<u>Will You Still Need Me:</u>
<u>Finding Friends, Love and Meaning as We Age</u>
Written by Angela Browne-Miller.
Foreword by Evacheska DeAngelis

<u>Raising Thinking Children and Teens:</u>
<u>Guiding Mental and Moral Development</u>
Written by Angela Browne-Miller.
Foreword by Evacheska DeAngelis.

<u>International Collection on Addictions</u>
Dr. Angela Browne-Miller, Editor.

<u>Violence and Abuse in Society:</u>
<u>Understanding a Global Crisis</u>
Dr. Angela Browne-Miller, Editor.

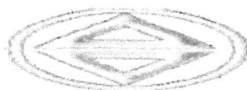

**metaterra®
publications**

Transcending Addiction and Other Afflictions, written by Angela Browne-Miller, is published by Metaterra® Publications for general distribution to readers all over the world. Metaterra® Publications is an independent publisher dedicated to the furthering of insight, wisdom, truth, learning, creativity, and perception. For other Metaterra® publications, both fiction and nonfiction, see the Metaterra Publications website:

http://www.Metaterra.com

www.ingramcontent.com/pod-product-compliance
Lightning Source LLC
Chambersburg PA
CBHW061731270326
41928CB00011B/2191